THERAPEUTIC CRAFTS

A practical approach

A practical approach

Cynthia Johnson, OTR
Kathy Lobdell, OTR
Jacqueline Nesbitt, OTR
Marjorie Clare

SLACK Incorporated, 6900 Grove Road, Thorofare, NJ 08086-9447

Editorial Director: Amy E. Drummond
Publisher: John H. Bond
Managing Editor: Debra L. Clarke

Photography by Todd Anderson, Minneapolis, Minnesota, 619-926-1593.

The procedures and practices described in this book should be implemented in a manner consistent with the professional standards set for the circumstances that apply in each specific situation. Every effort has been made to confirm the accuracy of the information presented and to correctly relate generally accepted practices. The authors, editor, and publisher cannot accept responsibility for errors or exclusions, outcomes of the application of the material presented herein, nor for injuries incurred while participating in the activities. There is no expressed or implied warranty of this book or information imparted by it.

Therapeutic crafts: a practical approach/Cindy Johnson...[et a1.].
p. cm.
Includes bibliographical references.
ISBN 1-55642-279-2 (alk. paper)
1. Handicraft--Therapeutic use. 2. Occupational therapy.
I. Johnson, Cindy
RM735-7H35T45 1996 96-27550
615.8'515--dc20 CIP

Printed in the United States of America

Published by: SLACK Incorporated
6900 Grove Road
Thorofare, NJ 08086 USA
Telephone: 609-848-1000
Fax: 609-853-5991

Contact SLACK Incorporated for further information about other books in this field or about the availability of our books from distributors outside the United States.

Last digit is print number: 10 9 8 7 6 5 4 3 2 1

Contents

Dedication

To Kate Wright, a wonderful mentor who taught me about life and art and to my children who taught me about life and fun.

CJ

With all my love to my wonderful husband who is supportive of anything I endeavor to do and to our children Nathan and Jeremy who taught me to keep on-going motivation for doing crafts by asking, "Can we do a project, Mom?"

KL

To my mother Nell Smidell Nesbitt who believes in my creative self and taught me how to improvise.

JN

To my parents for giving me life and an intensity to live it to the fullest; to my husband and three children for enriching my life immeasurably; and to all my brothers, sisters, and friends who are always there for me.

MC

To our very professional photographer, Todd Anderson, of Minneapolis. His work has enhanced our book.

To Paul "Tobster" Hanson of Burger Brothers who taught us the joy of fly tying.

A special thank you to Bekah Johnson and Elizabeth Henrikson who helped us prepare some of our samples.

Preface

Dear Fellow Therapists:

You may have longed for this very book. We've all felt the need for high-level tasks that could be done independently with illustrations and step-by-step written instructions.

This book can be used in several ways:

- A picture file that the patient/client can use to review to assist in activity selection.
- To provide a variety of choices available to clinicians.
- To allow the patient/client to function to his or her maximal level of independence.
- To maximize the therapist's use of time in the most cost-effective manner.
- Therapeutic implications and considerations are included to aid in project selec tion and treatment planning.

This book contains a wide variety of commonly used crafts, as well as some lenging high-level activities. The easy-to-understand treatment recommendations include appropriate patient groups, gradation of activities, any known precautio and a supply list.

Introduction

The current status of the medical community is one of fluctuation and change. The patient's shortened length of stay has affected treatment planning and influenced media used in the clinic settings. Therapists feel the time bind and while desiring to serve clients with quality care, increasing demands preclude time to investigate new media.

This volume meets the needs of increasing cost effectiveness and the expanding knowledge for the clinician with streamlined instructions and treatment components and photographs to spark the imagination.

Each of the 28 crafts presented is illustrated and analyzed to stimulate creativity for the client and therapist. The instructions are step-by-step. Treatment goals, activity components, precautions, and activity gradations are enumerated.

We believe this book will provide an invaluable resource to expand the therapist's effective use of media. This unique format allows independence for the therapist and the client, and the expanded repertoire enhances the possibilities for success in the finished product.

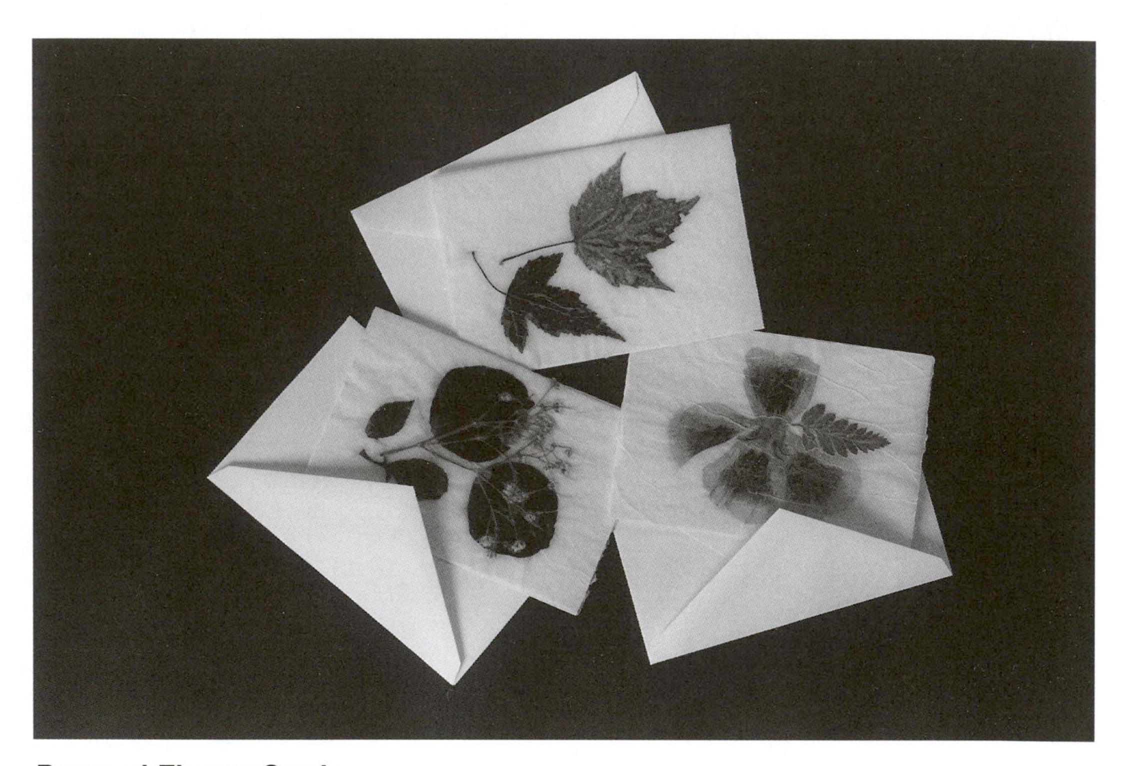

Pressed Flower Cards

Chapter 1

PRESSED FLOWER CARDS

Therapist Information for Pressed Flower Cards

ACTIVITY ANALYSIS

This project combines gardening as well as crafts. Flowers or leaves are first pressed, then used to make a parchment-appearing notecard, or can be framed. If flowers are already pressed, the project takes very little time to complete. It focuses on enhancing fine motor coordination and attention to detail. It may be useful in changing hand dominance.

This project may enhance performance in the following component areas:

Motor Components

- Fine motor abilities of the hand
- Hand dominance
- Strength

Cognitive Components

- Organizational abilities
- Problem-solving abilities
- Ability to plan
- Concentration
- Sequencing ability

Perceptual Components

- Eye-hand coordination
- Awareness of spatial relations
- Motor planning of hands and upper extremities

Emotional Components

- Independence
- Self-esteem

Social Components

- Sociability in new situations

Adaptations

- Position required—sitting upright or slightly reclined
- Allows for repetition of hand and finger motions
- Can be used for one-handed training with use of adaptive equipment
- High success rate
- Can vary from a structured to an unstructured activity
- Designs can incorporate some cultural values of an individual

GENERAL INFORMATION

1. Age—school age through adult
2. Cost—very inexpensive
3. Visual requirement—good visual acuity or corrected with glasses
4. Instructions can be given verbally, written, or through demonstration

SUPPLIES

- Tissues
- Notecards or paper
- Waxed paper
- Pressed flowers or leaves
- Small paint brush
- 12-inch ruler
- White glue
- Water
- Tweezer

PRECAUTIONS

This is generally a safe project. Pressed flowers or leaves will break, however, if not handled gently. This craft is not appropriate for clients who eat non-food items (PICA). This craft may be stressful for the small finger joints, as well as for carpal tunnel syndrome.

ACTIVITY GRADATION

Increase the number of flowers or leaves used for each card, or number of cards made.

NOTE This inexpensive craft can be used in coordination with the paper making activity included in this book. Many designs can be made using flowers, leaves, or a combination of both. These very attractive note cards can carry your personal messages to friends.

Client Information for Pressed Flower Cards

SUPPLIES

- Tissues
- Notecards or paper
- Waxed paper
- Pressed flowers or leaves
- Small paint brush
- 12-inch ruler
- White glue
- Water
- Tweezer

INSTRUCTIONS

1. Press flowers or leaves between pages of a book or in a commercial flower press until dry (about 5 to 7 days before beginning card project).
2. Select notecard or paper.
3. Cut piece of waxed paper larger than unfolded notecard or paper.
4. Choose pressed flowers or leaves for design and position on top of waxed paper.
5. Mix equal parts of glue and water.
6. Pull two-ply tissue gently apart into two sheets.
7. Put one thin sheet of tissue over design of flowers on waxed paper.
8. Brush glue on tissue carefully, starting on flowers or leaves, then move to edge of paper.

9. Let dry for at least half an hour.
10. With notecard underneath, tear waxed paper along edge of ruler to match size of card or paper.
11. Fold notecard and designed waxed paper together.

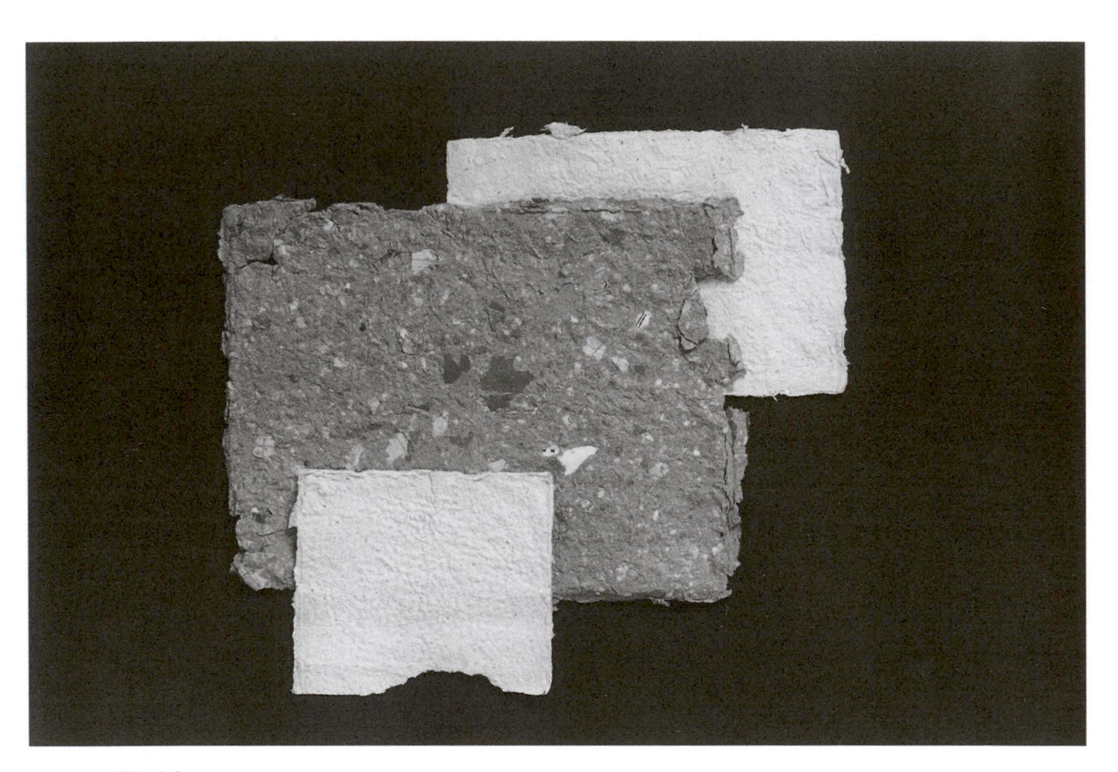

Paper Making

Chapter 2

PAPER MAKING

Therapist Information for Paper Making

ACTIVITY ANALYSIS

Paper making is an easy process and can be quite creative. It can be a first step in developing another craft project (i.e., collage or pressed flower cards). This is a relaxing task that does not require client's full attention during all stages of the process. There are some rote steps that would be appropriate for clients with attentional problems. This gross motor activity combines tactile input and finger strengthening. A good craft for visually impaired clients. All ages can participate and it is a great way to recycle all that junk mail.

This project may enhance performance in the following component areas:

Motor Components

- Fine motor abilities of the hand
- Hand dominance
- Use of hands bilaterally
- Strength in the upper extremity

Cognitive Components

- Sequencing ability
- Organizational abilities
- Problem-solving abilities
- Concentration

Perceptual Components

- Tactile awareness in the hands
- Motor planning of hands and upper extremities
- Awareness of neglected side

Emotional Components

- Release of negative feelings

- Expression of feelings—both negative and positive

Adaptations

- Position required—sitting and standing, could not be done from bed or semi-reclined position
- Allows for repetition of hand and finger motions
- Can be used for one-handed training, with use of adaptive equipment
- High success rate
- Can be done individually
- Can be adapted for a group

GENERAL INFORMATION

1. Age—teenager through adult
2. Cost—expensive if frames need to be purchased
3. Visual requirements—visual acuity is not required for this project. Blender operation could pose a safety problem for a blind client who has not been previously instructed in blender operations
4. Instructions can be given verbally, written, or through demonstration

SUPPLIES

- Paper to be recycled
- Blender
- Oblong container to put paper pulp in
- Old bath towel
- Clean newspaper
- Knife
- Heavy books or objects
- Purchased small wooden frame with screening attached

PRECAUTIONS

Blender operation may require supervision. Paper pulp will become moldy after 3 days and needs to be discarded. Because of potential for mold some respiratory patients may not be able to do this craft. No open hand wounds. May be stressful to small joints of the hand.

ACTIVITY GRADATION

Tear more than one sheet at a time to use for finger strengthening. Obtain special effects by adding different colors of paper, glitter, or paper punch-outs to pulp mixture.

NOTE This is a good craft for working out angry feelings. Tearing paper can help do this. Paper making is a good craft for environmentally aware citizens of the earth because it is direct recycling for old/used paper. Paper making can also be the first step in other craft ventures, such as collage art or card making.

Client Information for Paper Making

SUPPLIES

- Paper to be recycled
- Blender
- Oblong container to put paper pulp in
- Old bath towel
- Clean newspaper
- Knife
- Heavy books or objects
- Purchased small wooden frame with screening attached

INSTRUCTIONS

1. Select scrap paper, not metallic or plastic wrap (such as window envelopes).
2. Tear paper into 1-inch squares—four to five sheets.
3. Put into blender with approximately 4 cups of water.
4. With blender lid on, grind on low setting for approximately 10 seconds or until paper has turned to pulp.
5. Pour into oblong container.
6. Repeat steps 1 through 5, three times or until oblong container is filled to about 5 inches deep.
7. Stir pulp with hands to evenly distribute the pulp throughout the oblong container.

8. Put the screened frame into the water by going down one side of container and laying the frame on the bottom of the container.
9. With hands, brush water and pulp mixture around and over the screened frame to evenly cover the frame with paper pulp.
10. Carefully lift the screened frame straight up out of paper pulp mixture. This paper pulp will dry and become your newly made paper.
11. Allow the excess water to drain off through the bottom of the screen.
12. Lay frame on a flat surface until paper is fully dried on screen. This may take overnight.
13. To remove the dried paper from the screen, use fingers to gently loosen and lift the edges of the paper, then run the blade of a butter knife under the paper gently to lift it off the screen.

CORRECTING MISTAKES

If pulp on screen is not even in thickness, the thin spots will weaken the paper. If you notice that you have thin spots or holes, dump the paper pulp back into the container and restart the process. Use hands to agitate paper pulp in water so it flows over screen evenly.

CARE OF PROJECT

Use this paper, as you would any paper, for writing or for crafts; however, if you use a felt tip marker on new paper, it may bleed or run.

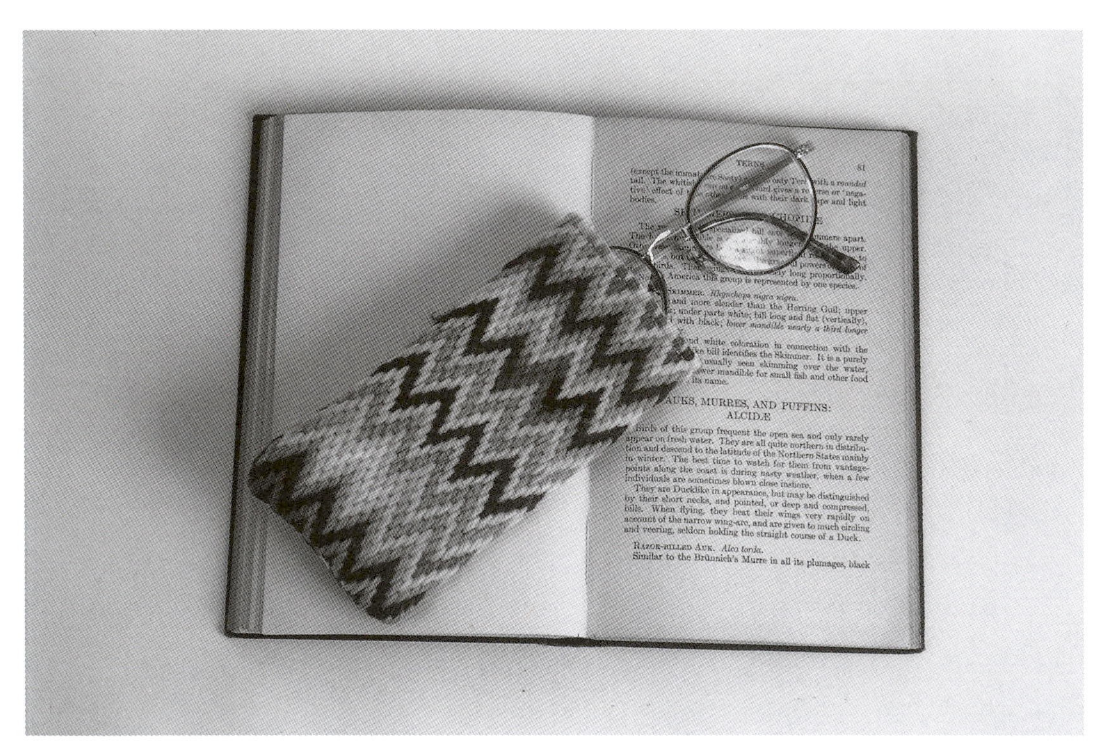

Bargello

Chapter 3

BARGELLO

Therapist Information for Bargello

ACTIVITY ANALYSIS

Bargello (long or flame stitch) has been done since needlework began, and this stitch is referred to by either of these names. The design can be worked quickly, is fun to do, and once the pattern is established it is a simple project. This needlecraft project uses yarn scraps or multi-colored yarns, making it a low-cost project. This is a gross motor activity for upper extremity strength. Fine motor components are also involved in holding the needle and doing the stitches. It is a good craft for changing dominance and can be done one-handed with adaptive equipment.

This project may enhance performance in the following component areas:

Motor Components

- Fine motor abilities of the hand
- Hand dominance
- Use of hands bilaterally
- Endurance

Cognitive Components

- Ability to plan
- Concentration
- Attention to task

Perceptual Components

- Eye-hand coordination
- Awareness of spatial relations
- Tactile awareness in the hands
- Motor planning of hands and upper extremities
- Constructional apraxia

Emotional Components

- Independence
- Self-esteem

Social Components

- Comfort level in group settings
- Sociability in new situations
- Ability to work alone

Adaptations

- Position required—sitting upright or reclining in bed
- Allows for repetition of hand and finger motions
- High success rate
- Can be done individually
- Can be used for one-handed training, with use of adaptive equipment

GENERAL INFORMATION

1. Age—teenager through adult
2. Cost—inexpensive
3. Visual requirements—good visual acuity or corrected by glasses
4. Instructions can be given verbally, written, or through demonstration

SUPPLIES

- Yarn
- Canvas (our project used 14 count)
- Needle
- Scissors
- Thimble

PRECAUTIONS

Precautions with sharp objects may need to be observed because of a sharp needle and scissors. This may be a difficult task for those with tremors or severe incoordination. Static hand position may be stressful to the small hand joints.

ACTIVITY GRADATION

This activity can be graded by varying the size of the project, the complexity of the design, or by using different yarn colors (rather than variegated).

NOTE Bargello is an easy needlepoint craft to learn. Once the pattern is established, it is easy to follow. You can use a wide variety of color combinations to match any decor. This can be a great leisure activity that will provide hours of relaxation. Bargello can be used as a pillow, chair seats covers, or eyeglass case for a smaller project.

Client Information for Bargello

SUPPLIES

- Yarn
- Canvas (our project used 14 count)
- Needle
- Scissors
- Thimble

INSTRUCTIONS

1. Mark a square on the canvas the same size as your project.

   Note: Leave a 1-inch border around all sides of your project.

2. At approximately half way down from the top of your project on the left edge, put your needle into the canvas and weave in/out (in a type of running stitch) for approximately 1 inch (Figure 3-1).

   Note: The first row of stitches determines the depth and variation of the points.

3. Start with running stitches and draw needle to front of canvas in first mesh of area to be worked.

4. The straight vertical stitch is worked from left to right over three threads, each succeeding stitch two threads higher than the preceding stitch until peak is reached.

5. Working downward on the right, repeat the same number of stitches that are on the left.

6. Continue alternating groups of stitches.

Figure 3-1

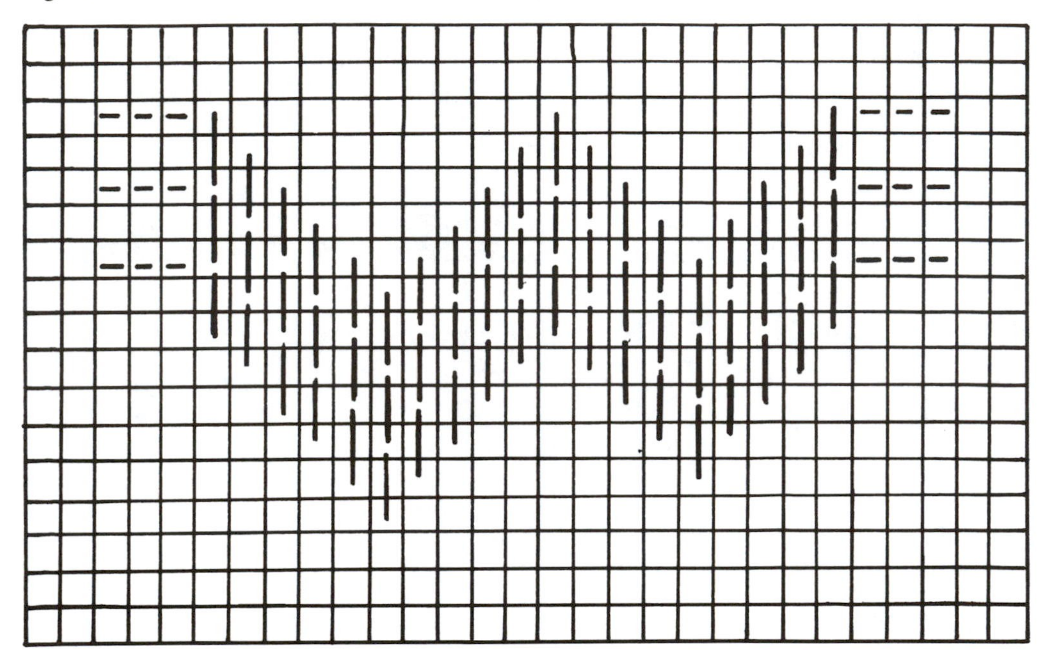

7. Continue with rows in various lengths of stitches until desired area is filled. To complete the top and bottom edges, fill in the empty triangles with rows of stitches.

CORRECTING MISTAKES

Pull out yarn back to point of error and resume stitching.

CARE OF PROJECT

Wash with a damp cloth, but do not submerge in water. Can be dry cleaned.

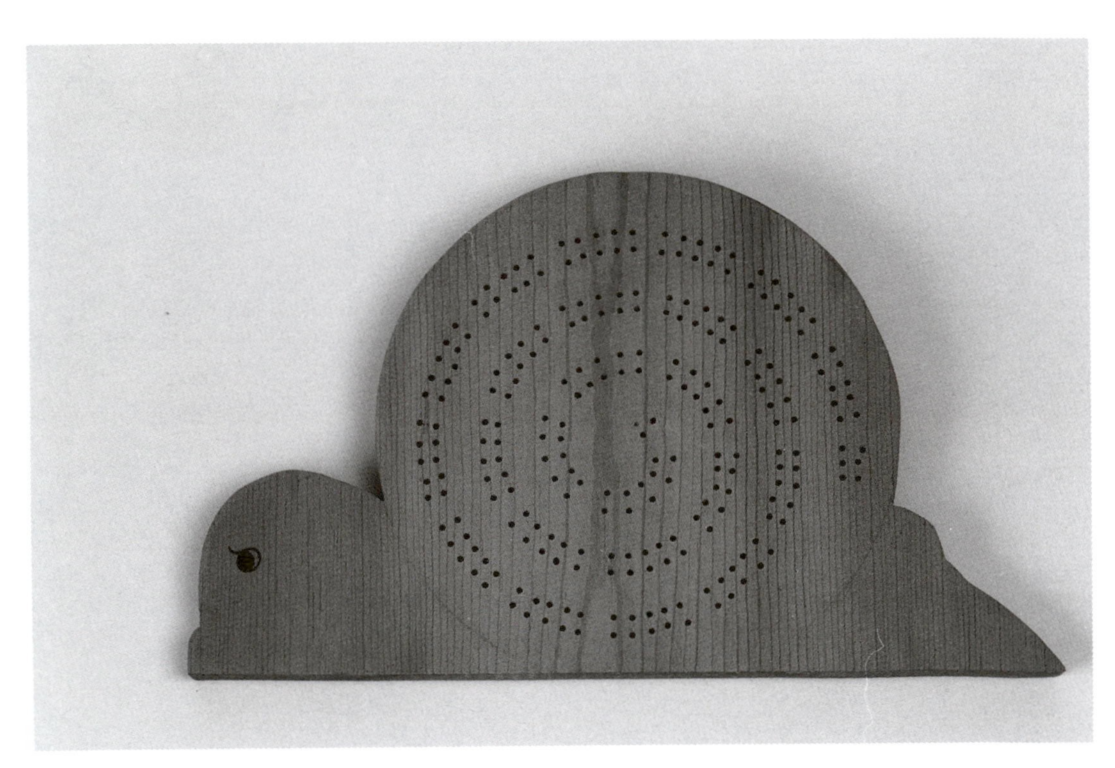

Snail Cribbage Board

Chapter 4

SNAIL CRIBBAGE BOARD

Therapist Information for Snail Cribbage Board

ACTIVITY ANALYSIS

This project can be graded easily according to a client's abilities. Use of power tools and planning/purchasing of all materials can greatly increase complexity of the task. It is structured in its pattern and directions, but choices can be allowed such as stain, color, and what to use for cribbage pegs. It uses strength of the upper extremity and trunk muscles. It's a very cognitive craft as attention to task is required.

Special Note: This activity is an excellent pre-vocational evaluation for safety and judgment with power tools.

This project may enhance performance in the following component areas:

Motor Component

- Fine motor abilities of the hand
- Coordination of the hand
- Use of hands bilaterally
- Endurance
- Strength of the upper extremity and trunk muscles

Cognitive Components

- Organizational abilities
- Problem-solving abilities
- Ability to plan
- Attention to task
- Sequencing ability
- Decision-making skills

Perceptual Components

- Eye-hand coordination
- Awareness of spatial relations

- Tactile awareness in the hands
- Motor planning of hands and upper extremities
- Constructional praxia

Emotional Components

- Independence
- Self-esteem

Social Components

- Ability to work alone

Adaptations

- Position required: upright, sitting, or standing
- May be done on incline board with weights used on sander or client

GENERAL INFORMATION

1. Age—teenager through adult
2. Cost—minimal
3. Visual requirements—good visual acuity or corrected with glasses
4. Instructions can be given verbally, written, or through demonstration

SUPPLIES

- 12 inches by 10 inches pine board
- Power band saw
- Power drill press
- Pattern
- Sand paper
- Graphite paper
- Stain
- Finish (varnish)
- Brush
- Cloths
- Safety glasses
- Purchased pegs or dowel to fit holes
- Black paint

PRECAUTIONS

This particular activity involves the use of power tools which can harm or mangle fingers. The therapist must remain vigilant while the client uses power tools. This is not a one-handed task and is not appropriate for clients that are highly impulsive or who have a severe field cut. Clients with respiratory problems may find this craft irritating due to sawdust and varnishes.

NOTE Card games are a pleasurable recreational activity and this project provides opportunity to create a cribbage board for yourself or a family member. This craft requires the use of power tools and can be stained or painted as chosen.

Client Information for Snail Cribbage Board

SUPPLIES

- 12 inches by 10 inches pine board
- Power band saw
- Power drill press
- Pattern
- Sand paper
- Graphite paper
- Stain
- Finish (varnish)
- Brush
- Cloths
- Safety glasses
- Purchased pegs or dowel to fit holes
- Black paint

INSTRUCTIONS

1. Trace pattern onto wood surface (Figure 4-1).
2. Cut with band saw along outside line.
3. Drill all hole markings using an electric drill press.
4. Sand all edges and surfaces.
5. Stain and finish according to directions on can of stain or finish.

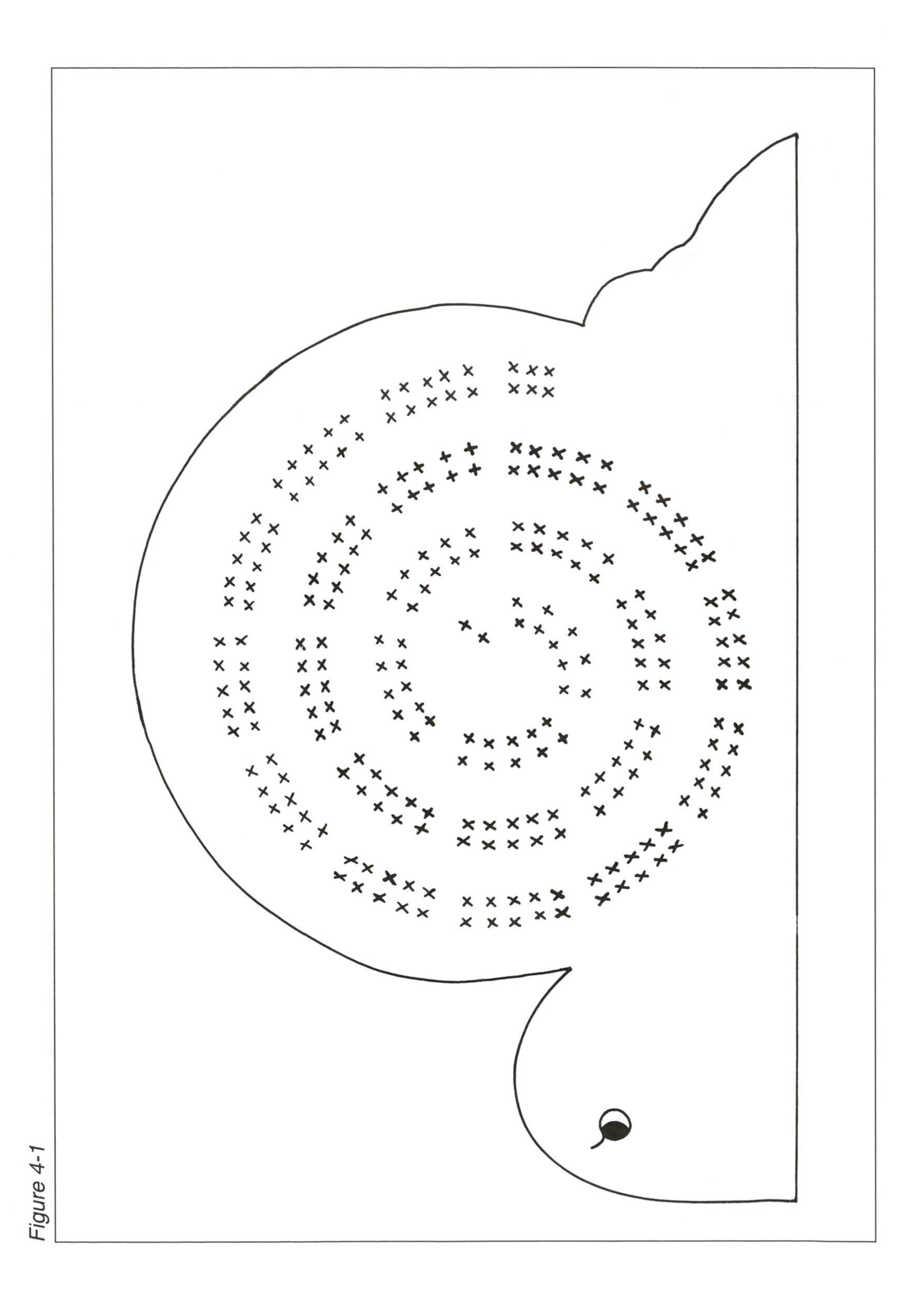

Figure 4-1

6. Buy pegs or cut pieces of dowel to fit holes.
7. Draw on an eye as shown in pattern or purchase eye-bead to finish project.

CORRECTING MISTAKES

Unable to correct cutting errors as wood is an uncorrectable medium.

CARE OF PROJECT

Can dust, do not immerse in water.

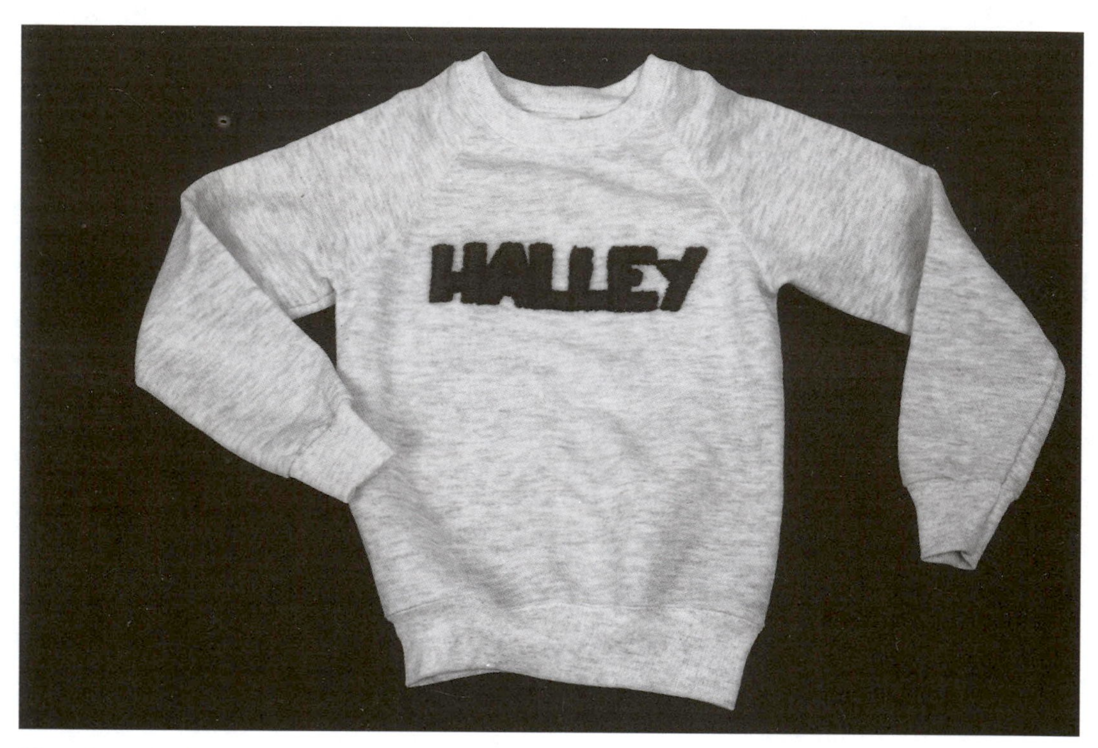

Needlepunch

Chapter 5

NEEDLEPUNCH

Therapist Information for Needlepunch

ACTIVITY ANALYSIS

Needlepunch is a craft activity that incorporates the use of a special punch and six-strand embroidery floss to complete a specific design. The design consists of small loops that appear solid when completed. This activity is a gross motor activity for upper extremity strengthening. There are also fine motor components in holding the needlepunch during punching. This craft may be useful in changing hand dominance or one-handed training with use of adaptive equipment.

This project may enhance performance in the following component areas:

Motor Components

- Fine motor abilities of the hand
- Coordination of the hand
- Hand dominance
- Use of hands bilaterally
- Endurance

Cognitive Components

- Organizational abilities
- Problem-solving abilities
- Ability to plan
- Concentration
- Attention to task
- Sequencing ability
- Decision-making skills

Perceptual Components

- Eye-hand coordination
- Spatial relations

- Tactile awareness of the hands
- Motor planning of hands and upper extremities

Emotional Components

- Independence
- Release of negative feelings

Social Components

- Responsibility
- Ability to work alone

Adaptations

- Position required—sitting upright or reclining in bed
- Allows for repetition of hand and finger motions
- Can be used for one-handed training, with use of adaptive equipment
- High success rate
- Design could incorporate some individual cultural values

GENERAL INFORMATION

1. Age—teenager through adult
2. Cost—moderate
3. Visual requirements—good visual acuity or corrected with glasses
4. Instructions can be given verbally, written, or through demonstration

SUPPLIES

- Tightly woven fabric (i.e., cotton)
- Transferable design
- Embroidery hoop to fit design
- Six-strand embroidery floss
- Needlepunch and threader
- Embroidery scissors
- Iron

PRECAUTIONS

Precautions with sharp objects may need to be observed when using needles and scissors. This project may be stressful to small hand joints.

ACTIVITY GRADATION

Vary complexity of design and design size.

NOTE Needlepunch can be used to decorate clothing, pillows, and pictures. Almost any simple design can be adapted to needlepunch. Centuries ago, needlepunch was done by the Russian people using bird wing bones or a piece of rolled tin. This is a good craft to do while relaxing in front of the television.

Client Information for Needlepunch

SUPPLIES

- Tightly woven fabric (i.e., cotton)
- Transferable design
- Embroidery hoop to fit design
- Six-strand embroidery floss
- Needlepunch and threader
- Embroidery scissors
- Iron

INSTRUCTIONS

Getting Ready to Punch

1. Practice is recommended before starting your design.
2. Transfer design to wrong side of fabric.
3. Stretch fabric in embroidery hoop until drum tight.
4. If just beginning, number one needle and one strand are recommended.

Threading Needlepunch

1. Adjust needle length using guide to vary length of loops in the finished product.

   Note: a) The eye of the needle and the knob to adjust needle should always be parallel to each other, b) 8-mm-needle-length was used in our design.
2. Insert needle threader, loop end first, through hollow needle of the punch.

3. Bring threader through handle and out top until threader loop is exposed. (Don't pull through all the way.)
4. Put floss through the loop about 20 to 30 inches.
5. Pull threader back through handle and out needle until the floss and threader come out through needle on punch.
6. Take threader and pull through eye of needle to thread floss.
7. Remove threader.
8. You are now ready to punch.

Punching

1. Start with about 2 inches of floss extended from the eye of the needle.
2. Brace hoop with hand, edge of table, or firm pillow in lap.
3. Hold needle in vertical position.
4. Push needle all the way into the wrong side of fabric until the fabric and plastic handle meet.
5. Pull up only to the surface of the fabric.
6. Drag across material and then insert for next stitch. Keep eye of the needle facing the last stitch or loop will not form properly.
7. Repeat steps 3 through 6 (on wrong side of cloth) until design is complete.
8. Cut loose strands to avoid accidentally pulling out your work.
9. Work design from outside to inside for best results.
10. Clip stray floss ends down to loop on right side of design.

CORRECTING MISTAKES

- Pull floss to remove unwanted stitches.
- Close hole in fabric by scraping fabric with a needle point.
- Repunch using new floss to avoid problems.

CARE OF PROJECT

Needlepunch is machine washable if washable materials are used. Washing often tightens up the fabric, holding the loops in better. For frequently washed items, use fabric glue on wrong side to secure needlepunching.

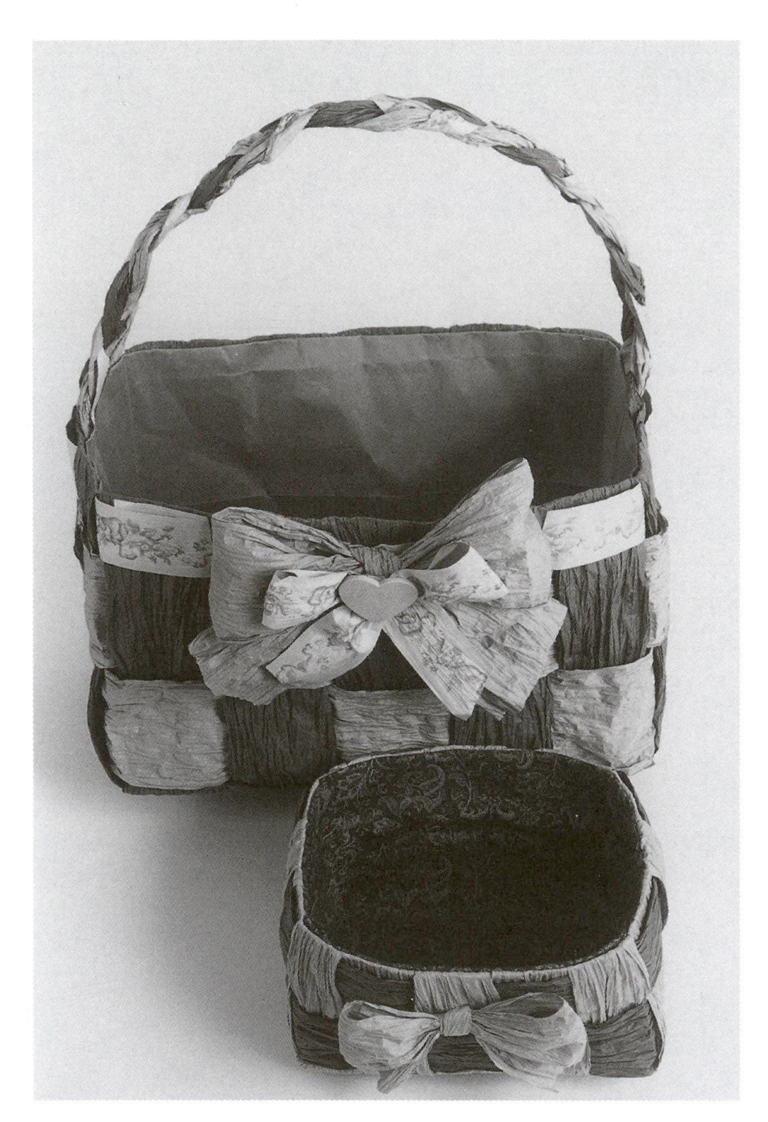

Paper Twist Basket

Chapter 6

PAPER TWIST BASKET

Therapist Information for Paper Twist Basket

ACTIVITY ANALYSIS

This fairly new craft is an excellent fine motor as well as gross motor activity, appropriate for a group or individuals. Exclusive of the glue gun, this is a low-cost project with very satisfying results. It requires 2–3 hours to complete and can be varied by color and size. There is an emphasis for thumb/finger opposition while using scissors and in handling paper twist.

This project may enhance performance in the following component areas:

Motor Components

- Fine motor abilities of the hand
- Gross coordination of the hand/arm
- Hand dominance
- Use of the hands bilaterally
- Endurance
- Strength

Cognitive Components

- Organizational abilities
- Problem-solving abilities
- Ability to plan
- Concentration
- Attention to task
- Sequencing ability

Perceptual Components

- Eye-hand coordination
- Awareness of spatial relations
- Tactile awareness in the hands

- Motor planning of hands and upper extremities
- Constructional apraxia

Emotional Components

- Independence
- Self-esteem

Social Components

- Comfort level in group settings
- Sociability with new situations
- Ability to work alone

Adaptations

- Position required—sitting upright
- Allows for repetition of hand and finger motion
- Can be done individually
- Can be adapted for a group

GENERAL INFORMATION

1. Age—teenager through adult
2. Cost—inexpensive (excluding glue gun)
3. Visual requirements—good visual acuity or corrected with glasses
4. Instructions can be given verbally, written, or through demonstration

SUPPLIES

- Two large grocery bags
- Eight yards main color paper twist (untwisted)
- Six yards second color paper twist (untwisted)
- Glue gun/glue stick
- Scissors

PRECAUTIONS

Precautions need to be observed because of scissors and hot glue gun. Hot glue gun can burn fingers. Clients will need to be proficient in using the gule gun or the gluing can be done for them. Paper cuts may also be a problem. May be contraindicated for clients with carpal tunnel syndrome or problems with the small joints of the hand.

ACTIVITY GRADATION

Size of bag (i.e., grocery bag, lunch bag), ribbon size and color, additions (i.e., bows).

NOTE This fairly new craft will help to improve fine motor skills. It is inexpensive and can become a life-long hobby. You can individualize by adding bows, changing colors, and changing handles. It can be made in grocery bag-size or lunch bag-size.

Client Information for Paper Twist Basket

SUPPLIES

- Two large grocery bags
- Eight yards main color paper twist (untwisted)
- Six yards second color paper twist (untwisted)
- Glue gun/glue stick
- Scissors

INSTRUCTIONS

1. On one grocery bag measure 6 inches and 5½ inches from the bottom of the bag and draw lines around entire bag at these measurements.
2. Cut at the 6-inch line across the bag.
3. Fold edge to inside of bag at 5½-inch line.
4. Cut second bag at 5½-inch marking across bag. This bag will go inside the first bag.
5. Cut eight strips, 23 inches long, and three strips 29 inches long, of main color.
6. Glue three 29 inch strips across long side of first bag, from end to end and underneath bag (Figure 6-1).
7. Glue five 23-inch strips from side to side and underneath bag. Glue end of each strip to inside of bag. Weave bottom (Figure 6-2).
8. Cut three 42-inch strips of second color.
9. Weave three strips of the second color in and out all the way around the basket, glueing at the ends only, when under first color strip.

10. To make handle, braid remaining three 23-inch strips of main color. Glue to ends of bag and near top of bag.
11. Put second bag inside of first and glue inside around top of bag. This covers all construction work and finishes the project.
12. A bow may be made of extra paper twist and glued on where preferred.

CORRECTING MISTAKES

Pieces can be pulled apart before glue dries and reglued.

CARE OF PROJECT

Do not immerse in water, but dry dust.

Figure 6-1

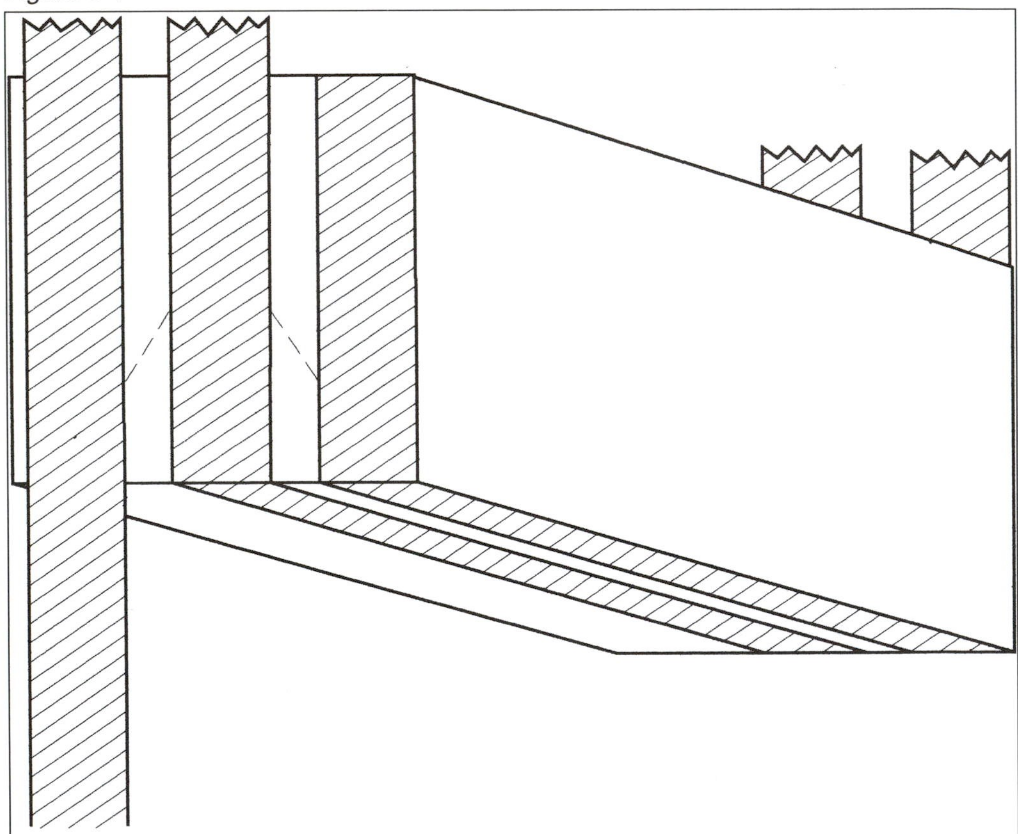

Figure 6-2

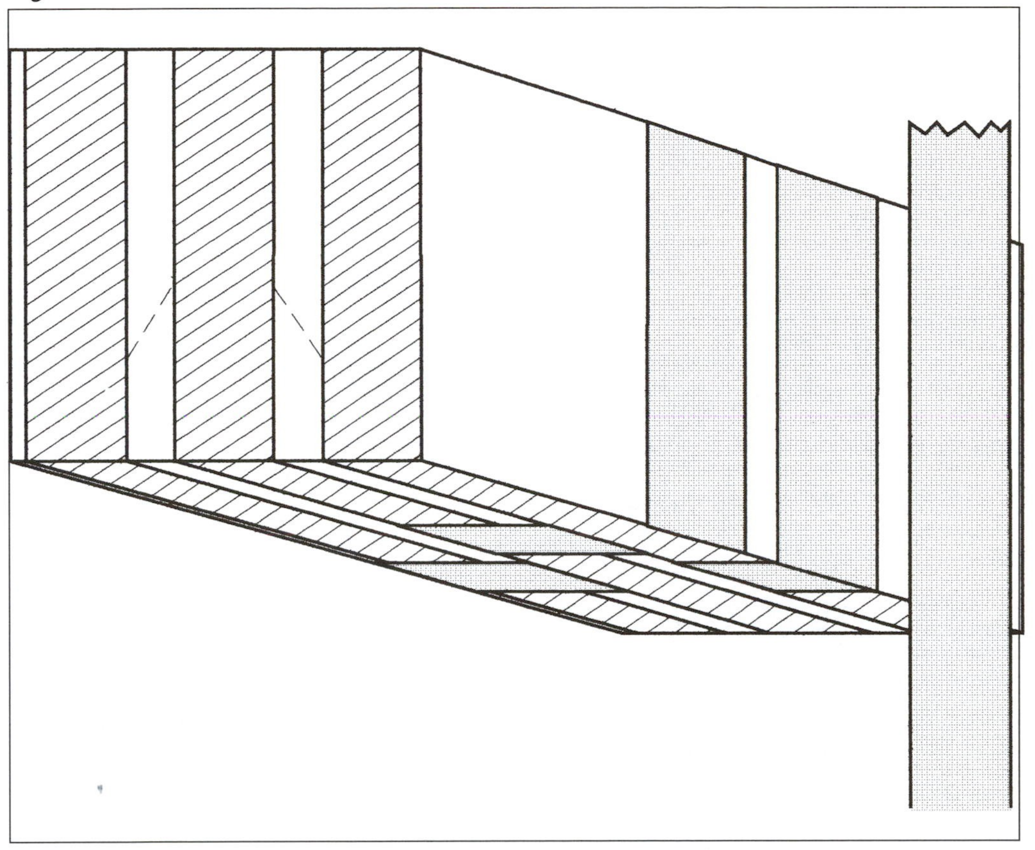

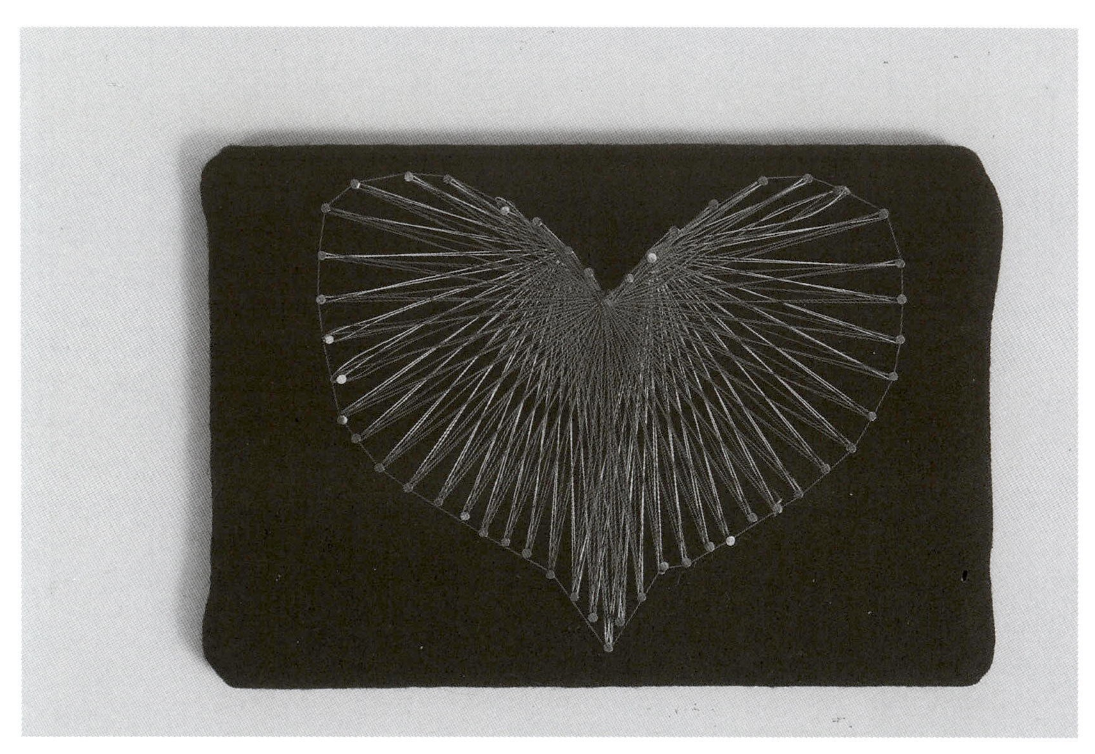

String Art

Chapter 7

STRING ART

Therapist Information for String Art

ACTIVITY ANALYSIS

This project combines string or yarn and nails to create intricate designs that are bright and colorful. The design is accomplished by wrapping string/yarn around the nails according to a specific pattern. It is relatively inexpensive. It requires close attention to detail, and is a bilateral fine motor activity.

This project may enhance performance in the following component areas:

Motor Components

- Fine motor abilities of the hand
- Coordination of the hand/arm
- Use of hands bilaterally
- Strength

Cognitive Components

- Organizational abilities
- Problem-solving abilities
- Ability to plan
- Concentration
- Attention to task
- Sequencing ability

Perceptual Components

- Eye-hand coordination
- Awareness of spatial relations
- Tactile awareness in the hands
- Motor planning of hands and upper extremities

Emotional Components

- Independence
- Self-esteem

Social Components

- Ability to work alone
- Comfort level in group settings

Adaptations

- Position required—sitting upright or reclining in bed
- Allows for repetition of hand and finger motions
- Can be done independently
- Design could incorporate some individual cultural values

GENERAL INFORMATION

1. Age—school age through adult
2. Cost—inexpensive
3. Visual requirements—good visual acuity or corrected with glasses
4. Instructions can be given verbally, written, or through demonstration

SUPPLIES

- Board, 3/4 inch thick, 5 inches by 7 inches
- Fabric for covering board (i.e., felt/burlap), 7 inches by 9 inches
- Brads (50 needed) 1/2 inch long with flat heads
- Thread, three small spools of different colors (example uses pink, purple, red)
- Stapler
- Hammer
- Ruler
- Scissors
- Glue
- Optional: awl (for hole starting), pliers (straightening brads or holding brads for nailing)

PRECAUTIONS

Precautions using sharp objects may need to be observed because of need for scissors. General precautions are needed for hammer and nail usage if the patient is impulsive. Infection control precautions are needed if puncture or bruising are concerns for client. Project may be difficult for clients with tremors, extreme incoordination, or may be contraindicated for clients with carpal tunnel syndrome or involvement of small hand joints.

ACTIVITY GRADATION

This activity can be graded by varying the size of brads (bigger or smaller), using thicker yarns, and by using a more complex design.

NOTE String art using colored threads can be intricate, beautiful, and a fascinating form of art. More advanced crafters can create their own designs. Following the specific pattern is the key to success with string art.

Client Information for String Art

SUPPLIES

- Board, 3/4 inch thick, 5 inches by 7 inches
- Fabric for covering board (i.e., felt/burlap), 7 inches by 9 inches
- Brads (50 needed) 1/2 inch long with flat heads
- Thread, three small spools of different colors (example uses pink, purple, red)
- Stapler
- Hammer
- Ruler
- Scissors
- Glue
- Optional: awl (for hole starting), pliers (straightening brads or holding brads for nailing)

INSTRUCTIONS

1. Select a board and cover it with felt, stapling the edge of the fabric to back side of the board.
2. Center and tape down the pattern over the felt board.
3. Pound the brads into the dots indicated on the pattern.
4. Use pliers to make brads a uniform height and angle to the board.
5. Tie first color choice to nail A (Figure 7-1).
6. Wrap thread/yarn back around nail 1.
7. Wrap around nail A.

8. Wrap thread/yarn back around nail 1.
9. Wrap back around nail A.
10. Continue wrapping thread/yarn consecutively until you reach nail 23.
    Note: Always wrap in the same direction so pattern looks organized.
11. End at nail A and tie off thread/yarn.
12. Put a dot of glue on the end to secure it firmly to brad.
13. Tie first color choice to nail B.
14. Wrap thread/yarn around nail 24.
15. Wrap thread/yarn around nail B.
16. Continue wrapping thread/yarn consecutively until you get to nail 40.
17. Go back to nail B and tie off thread/yarn.
18. Put a dot of glue on the end to secure it firmly to brad.
19. The first layer of the heart pattern is now complete.
20. Tie second color choice to nail C.
21. Wrap thread/yarn around nail 1.
22. Wrap thread/yarn around nail C.
23. Continue wrapping your thread/yarn consecutively until you get to nail 23.
24. Go back to nail C and tie off thread/yarn.
25. Put a dot of glue on the end to secure it firmly to brad.
26. Tie second color choice to nail D.
27. Wrap thread/yarn around nail 24.
28. Wrap thread/yarn back around nail D.
29. Continue wrapping thread/yarn consecutively until you get to nail 45.
30. Go back to nail D and tie off.
31. Put a dot of glue on end to secure it firmly to brad.
32. Tie third color choice to nail E.
33. Wrap thread/yarn around nail 1.

Figure 7-1

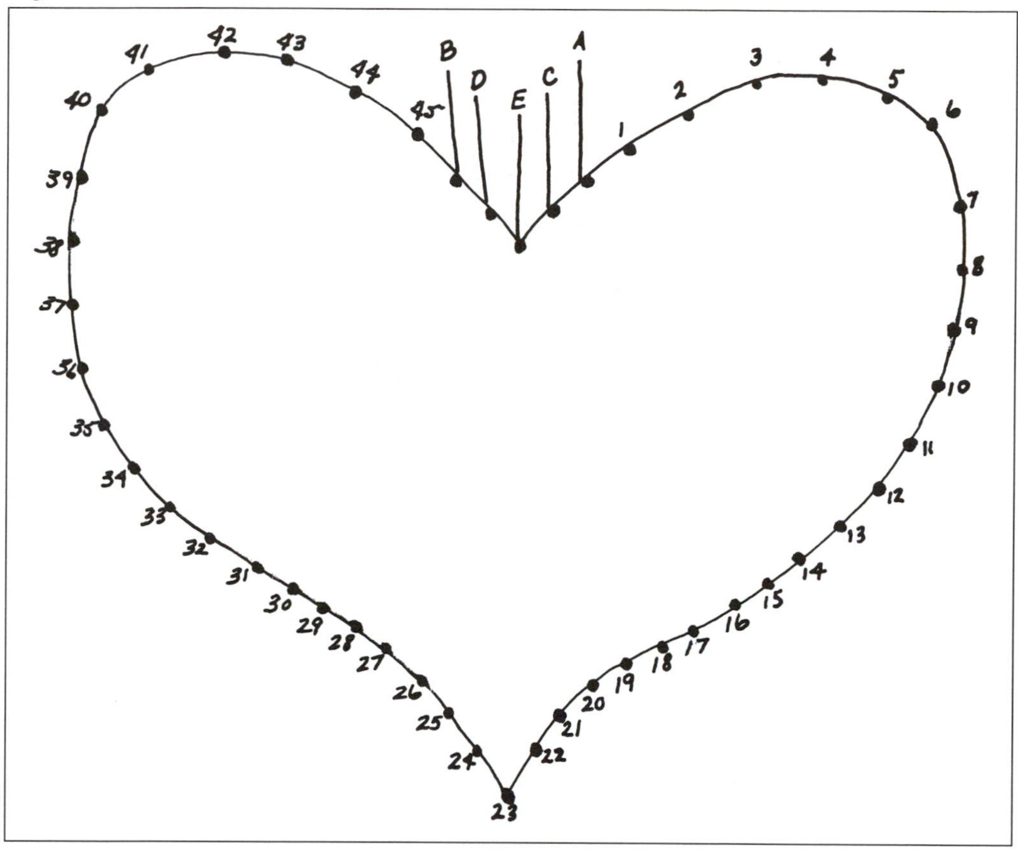

34. Wrap thread/yarn back around nail E.
35. Continue wrapping thread/yarn consecutively until you get to nail 45.
36. Tie off at nail E.
37. Put a dot of glue on end to secure firmly to brad.
38. Use tip of finger to raise all threads to top of brads.
39. Remove pattern carefully, so as not to pull out nails or dislodge threads.

CORRECTING MISTAKES

Unwrap thread/yarn back to point of error and restart wrapping.

CARE OF PROJECT

This project is delicate, so dust carefully; it is not washable.

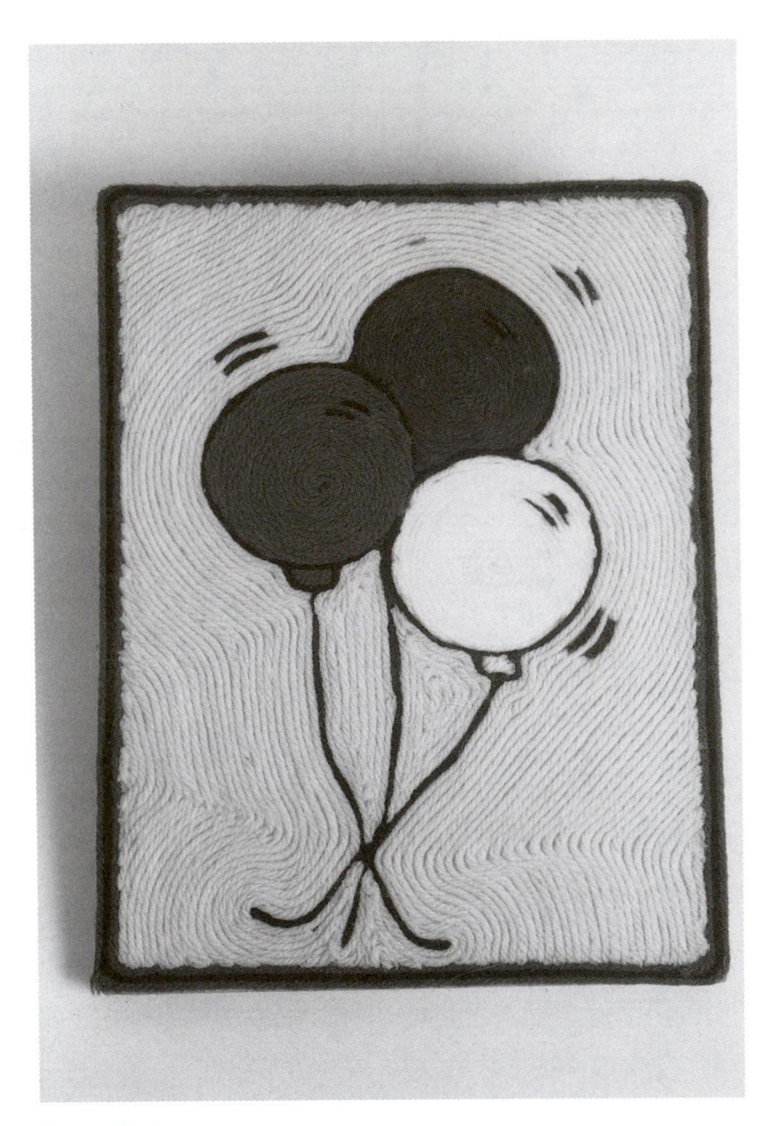

Yarn Picture

Chapter 8

YARN PICTURE

Therapist Information for Yarn Picture

ACTIVITY ANALYSIS

This is an excellent project in which to use scraps of yarn, macrame cord, jute, twine, and wood—making it a low-cost project. This is a relatively simple project, but still allows for some gradability. It is appropriate for young and old alike. The time needed to complete this project varies with size and design. It incorporates fine motor coordination with visual perceptual skills. There is also a strong tactile component.

This project may enhance performance in the following component areas:

Motor Component

- Fine motor abilities of the hand
- Coordination of the hand/arm
- Hand dominance
- Use of hands bilaterally

Cognitive Components

- Organizational abilities
- Problem-solving abilities
- Ability to plan
- Concentration
- Attention to task

Perceptual Components

- Eye-hand coordination
- Awareness of spatial relations
- Tactile awareness in the hands
- Motor planning of hands and upper extremities

Emotional Components

- Independence
- Self-esteem

Social Components

- Comfort level in group settings
- Sociability with new situations
- Ability to work alone

Adaptations

- Position required—sitting upright or reclining in bed
- Allows for repetition of hand and finger motions
- Can be used for one-handed training, with use of adaptive equipment
- High success rate
- Can be done individually
- Can be adapted for a group
- Design could incorporate some cultural values of an individual

GENERAL INFORMATION

1. Age—preschool through adult
2. Cost—minimal
3. Visual—good visual acuity needed or corrected with glasses
4. Instructions can be given verbally, written, or through demonstration

SUPPLIES

- Scraps of yarn or twine (any thickness)
- Pattern of choice
- Hard backing (cardboard)
- Tacky glue
- Scissors
- Tongue depressors or craft sticks
- Permanent marker
- Carbon paper

PRECAUTIONS

Scissors are needed. Standard precautions should be observed.

ACTIVITY GRADATION

Vary size of project or design. Use various thickness of yarn/twine within the same project.

NOTE This is a relatively simple project that is appropriate for young and old alike. It can use up supplies of leftover yarn. You will find it a relaxing project.

Client Information for Yarn Picture

SUPPLIES

- Scraps of yarn or twine (any thickness)
- Pattern of choice
- Hard backing (cardboard)
- Tacky glue
- Scissors
- Tongue depressors or craft sticks
- Permanent marker
- Carbon paper

INSTRUCTIONS

1. Trace pattern onto backing using carbon paper (Figure 8-1).

   Note: a) If design is on a piece of paper, it can be glued directly onto backing, b) Simple designs produce the best results.

2. Use the felt marker to go over the lines to make them easier to see and follow.
3. Use the brush to spread the glue onto one section of the design at a time, beginning in the center and working toward the edges.
4. Cut a length of yarn.
5. Press the yarn onto the tacky glue surface.
6. Continue steps 3 through 5 until the design is complete.

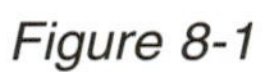

Figure 8-1

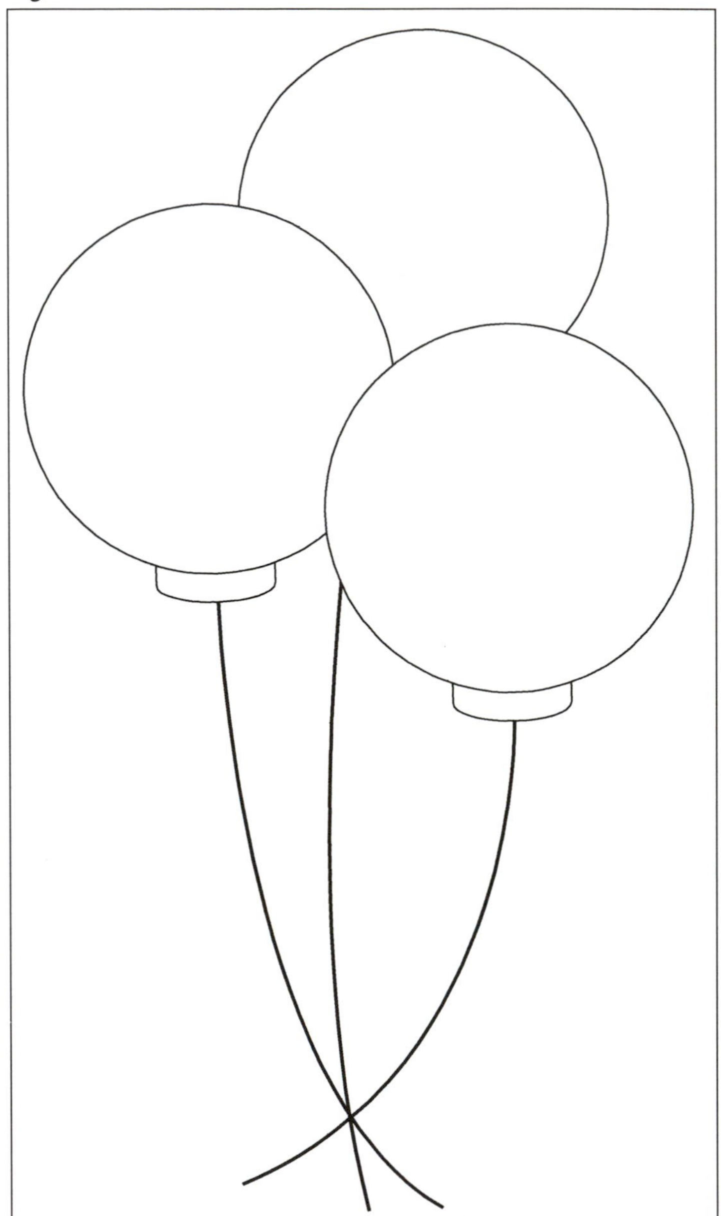

CORRECTING MISTAKES

If glue is wet, you can rearrange the yarn. If glue is dry, the pattern is established and cannot be rearranged.

CARE OF PROJECT

Can be dusted, but do not immerse in water.

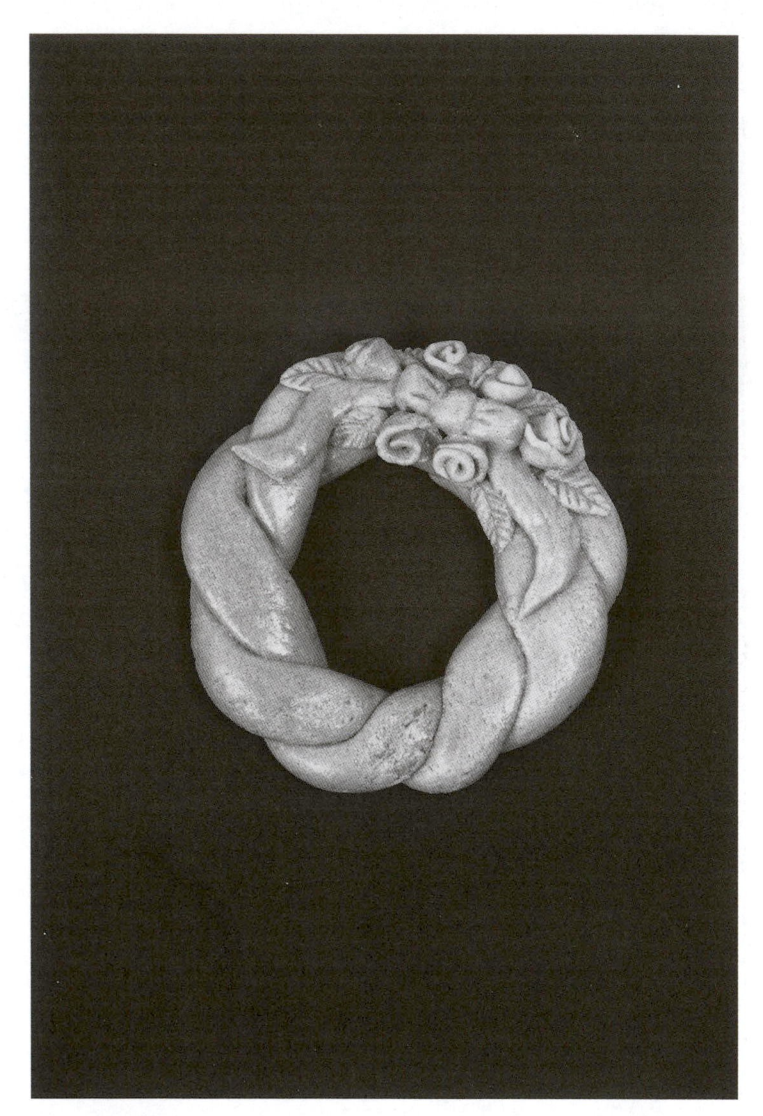

Dough Art

Chapter 9

DOUGH ART

Therapist Information for Dough Art

ACTIVITY ANALYSIS

This project can be done as a group task, just double the recipe. Each person can make his or her own sculpture or work on a larger group project. This dough is non-toxic, can be used with all ages, and allows for maximum creativity. This is a good craft for people who are visually impaired and have high tactile stimulation. It uses many of the upper extremity muscle groups. This project may enhance performance in the following component areas:

Motor Components

- Fine motor abilities of the hand
- Hand dominance
- Use of hands bilaterally
- Endurance
- Strength

Cognitive Components

- Concentration
- Attention to task
- Sequencing ability
- Decision-making skills

Perceptual Components

- Eye-hand coordination
- Tactile awareness in the hands
- Motor planning of hands and upper extremities

Emotional Components

- Independence
- Self-esteem

- Allows for release of negative feelings

Social Components
- Comfort level in group settings
- Sociability in new settings
- Ability to work alone

Adaptations
- Position required—sitting upright or standing
- Allows for repetition of hand and finger motions
- Can be unilateral with use of adaptive equipment
- High success rate
- Can vary from a structured to an unstructured activity
- Can be done individually
- Can be adapted for a group
- Design can incorporate some cultural values of an individual

GENERAL INFORMATION

1. Age—child to adult
2. Cost—minimal
3. Visual requirements—good visual skills are helpful, but not necessary
4. Instructions can be given verbally, written, or through demonstration

SUPPLIES

- Scraps of yarn or twine (any thickness)
- Pattern of choice
- Hard backing (cardboard)
- Tacky glue
- Scissors
- Tongue depressors or craft sticks
- Permanent marker
- Carbon paper

PRECAUTIONS

Precaution with sharp objects is necessary if using knives; however, plastic knives or other plastic utensils can be used instead. Store extra dough in refrigerator. Salt can be drying to skin; plastic gloves may be helpful. It is difficult to do the whole process in a bed rest situation.

ACTIVITY GRADATIONS

Project can be specific in what is to be made or allow for client's own creativity. More elaborate sculptures can be created by adding many dimensions (i.e., roses, bows), painting the project after it is dry, or altering the amount of dough used. The project can be done tactility with clients with visual impairments.

NOTE This is an easy medium to make and can be used to build anything your imagination can design. We chose a wreath design for our sample, but your choices are unlimited. Anything you can make from traditional clay, excluding cookware, can be made with dough art. After a project is dry, you can paint or varnish as desired.

Client Information for Dough Art

SUPPLIES

- Scraps of yarn or twine (any thickness)
- Pattern of choice
- Hard backing (cardboard)
- Tacky glue
- Scissors
- Tongue depressors or craft sticks
- Permanent marker
- Carbon paper

INSTRUCTIONS

1. In a large bowl, combine flour, salt, and water.
2. Mix well with spoon then knead dough with hands.

   Note: Dough should be pliable, not sticky or crumbly. If it is sticky, add small amounts of flour; if crumbly, add small amounts of water.
3. Roll out a handful of dough with hands to make a 12-inch rope.
4. Repeat step 3 so you will have two equal lengths of rope (Figure 9-1).
5. Cross two ropes in the middle.
6. Twist beginning from center until all 12 inches are twisted together (Figure 9-2).

7. Lay twisted ropes in a circle.
8. Press ends together.

   Note: Moistening the ends may help them stick together.
9. Add decorations described below by using ordinary household tools.

- Roses are made by forming a flat small ribbon of dough. Roll up ribbon with fingertips into rose buds and attach to wreath.
- Leaves are cut from flattened dough with a knife. Press the leaves gently into the wreath surface. Score veins into leaf.

Figure 9-1

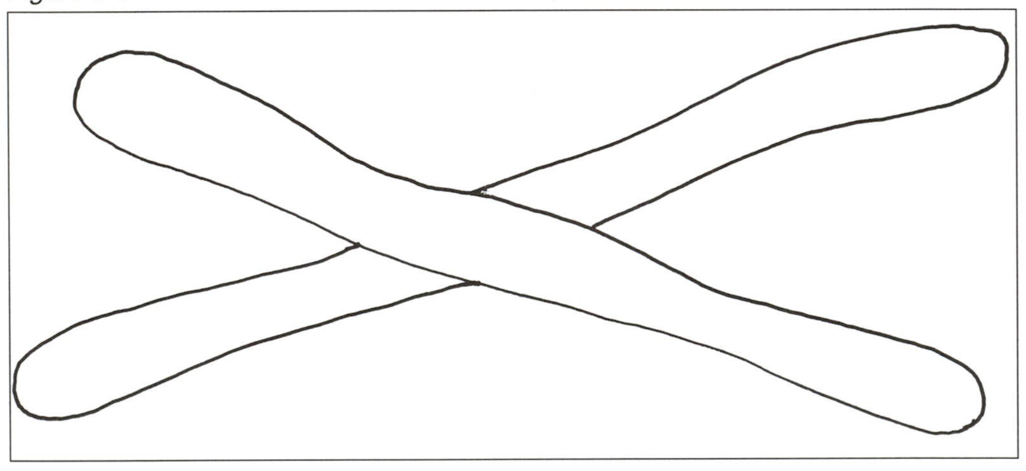

Figure 9-2

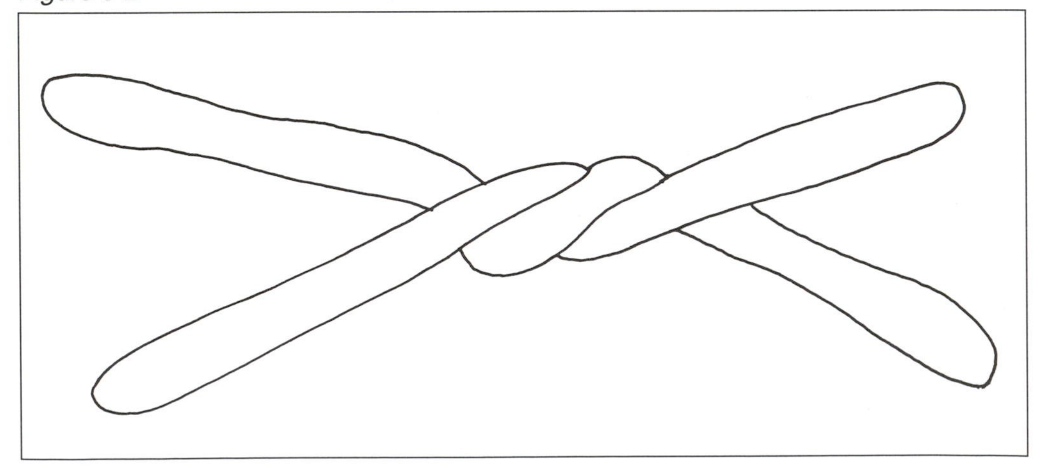

- Ribbons are made from flattened dough (as shown in picture) that has been cut. Lay the ribbon onto the wreath, press gently. Fold over end of the ribbon for a bow. Press in the middle and score with knife as shown in picture.

10. The project can air dry for several days or can be dried in an oven as follows; however do not vary the schedule:

    150°for first hour

    175° for second hour

    200° for third hour

    250° for fourth hour

    Note: We have found that oven drying is preferable.

CORRECTING MISTAKES

While dough is still wet, knead dough again and start over. A small amount of water can be added to make dough more pliable.

CARE OF PROJECT

Dust with dry cloth. Do not immerse in water.

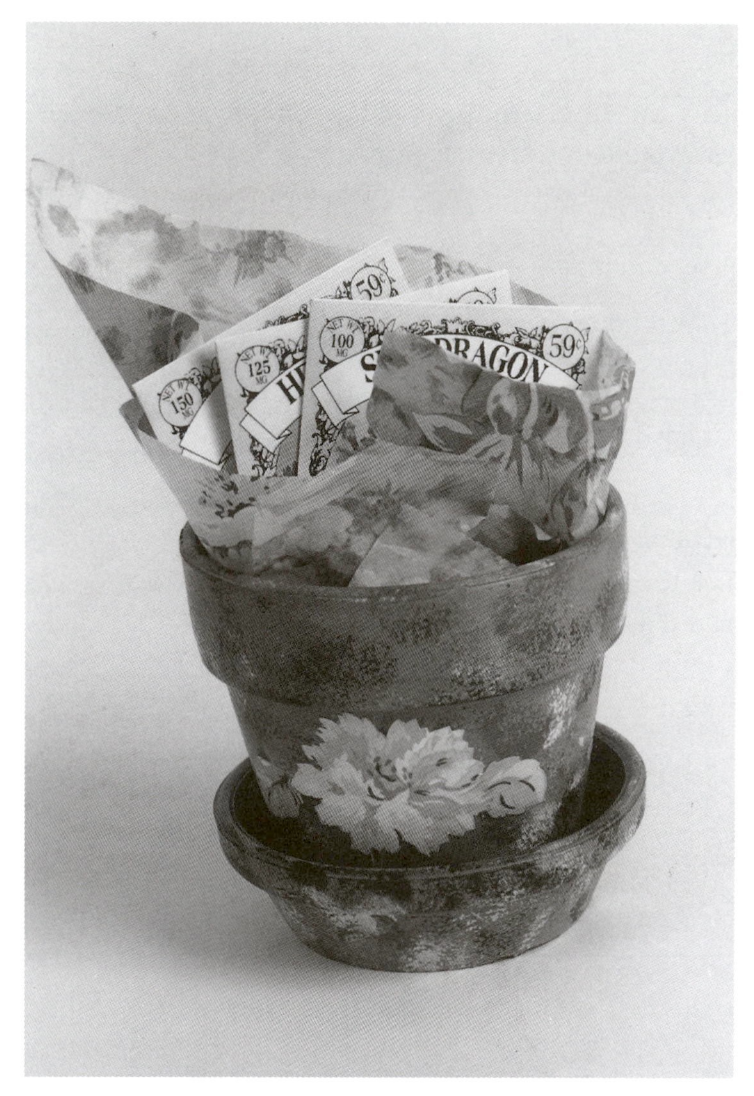

Decoupage/Sponge Paint Flower Pot

Chapter 10

DECOUPAGE/SPONGE PAINT FLOWER POT

Therapist Information for Decoupage/Sponge Paint Flower Pot

ACTIVITY ANALYSIS

This project combines several types of crafts and incorporates a greater number of steps in the process. There are several general choices to be made with this project (i.e., number of colors used, types and numbers of pictures, finishes). It can portray a client's individuality or become a group project if a large-size pot is chosen. This is a gross grasp project that does not require precision.

This project may enhance performance in the following component areas:

Motor Components

- Fine motor abilities of the hand
- Hand dominance
- Use of hands bilaterally
- Endurance

Cognitive Components

- Organizational abilities
- Problem-solving abilities
- Ability to plan
- Concentration
- Attention to task
- Sequencing ability
- Decision-making skills

Perceptual Components

- Eye-hand coordination

- Awareness of spatial relations
- Motor planning of the hands and upper extremities

Emotional Components

- Independence
- Self-esteem

Social Components

- Comfort level in group settings
- Ability to work alone

Adaptations

- Position required—sitting upright or standing
- Allows for repetition of hand and finger motions
- Can be unilateral with use of adaptive equipment
- High success rate
- Can vary from a structured to an unstructured activity
- Can be done individually
- Can be adapted for a group
- Design can incorporate some cultural values of an individual

GENERAL INFORMATION

1. Age—child to adult
2. Cost—minimal to moderate
3. Visual requirement—good visual acuity needed for design cut out and placement, however, not needed for decoupage portion or sponge painting
4. Instructions can be given verbally, written, or through demonstration

SUPPLIES

- 4-inch clay pot and base
- Scrap wallpaper or wrapping paper with designs that can be cut out
- Decoupage
- Paint brush
- Scissors
- Three colors of acrylic paint
- Small, rounded sponge

PRECAUTIONS

Precautions with sharp objects are necessary when using scissors for cutting out design. Not advisable for clients on bed rest.

ACTIVITY GRADATIONS

Design can be chosen and cut out for client. Paints can be chosen or therapist can paint the pot prior to session. The pot can be painted one color first to add another step to the process to work on organizational and planning skills.

NOTE This project can be used as a container for your favorite plant or small gift. Several paint colors can be sponged onto a terra cotta or painted flower pot. Color choice and picture used to decoupage can express your creativity.

Client Information for Decoupage/Sponge Paint Flower Pot

SUPPLIES

- 4-inch clay pot and base
- Scrap wallpaper or wrapping paper with designs that can be cut out
- Decoupage
- Paint brush
- Scissors
- Three colors of acrylic paint
- Small, rounded sponge

INSTRUCTIONS

1. Squeeze small amount of three colors of paint next to each other onto one plate.
2. Dip small sponge across all three colors.
3. Dab sponge on clay pot in a random pattern covering all of the pot and base.
4. Allow to dry completely before starting decoupage process.
5. Choose a picture from wallpaper or wrapping paper that you find pleasing and that fits onto the clay pot.

6. Cut out picture or design.
7. Paint decoupage finish onto the back of the picture or design using a paint brush.
8. Place picture or design onto surface of clay pot and press firmly into place trying not to wrinkle picture.
9. Paint decoupage finish over picture or design or paint over the whole pot if desired.
10. Allow to dry.
11. If you put finish all over the clay pot, also put the finish over the base for a more completed project.

CARE OF PROJECT

Do not immerse in water. Dust with soft cloth.

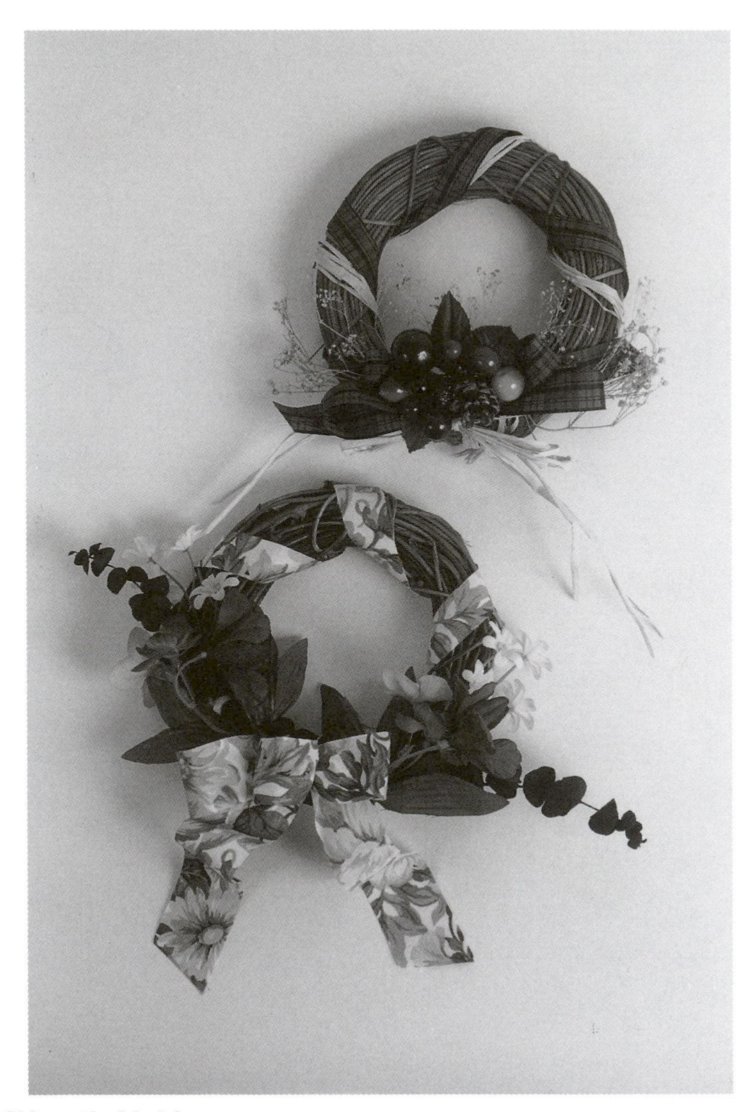

Wreath Making

Chapter 11

WREATH MAKING

Therapist Information for Wreath Making

ACTIVITY ANALYSIS

Wreath making is a popular craft that can allow for creativity and provide a sense of self-esteem in a short amount of time. A group task could be done around a central theme such as holiday wreaths. This is a gross motor activity for upper extremity strengthening and includes fine motor components when doing the detail work.

This project may enhance performance in the following component areas:

Motor Components

- Fine motor abilities of the hand
- Coordination of the hand/arm
- Hand dominance
- Use of hands bilaterally
- Endurance
- Strength

Cognitive Components

- Organizational abilities
- Problem-solving abilities
- Ability to plan
- Concentration
- Attention to task
- Sequencing ability
- Decision-making skills

Perceptual Components

- Eye-hand coordination
- Awareness of spatial relations
- Motor planning of hands and upper extremities

- Tactile awareness in the hands

Emotional Components
- Independence
- Self-esteem

Social Components
- Comfort level in group settings
- Sociability in new situations

Adaptations
- Position required—sitting upright or standing
- Allows for repetition of the hand and finger motion
- Can be unilateral with use of adaptive equipment
- High success rate
- Can vary from a structured to an unstructured activity
- Can be done individually
- Can be adapted for a group
- Design could incorporate some individual cultural values

GENERAL INFORMATION

1. Age—teenager to adult
2. Cost—minimal to expensive depending on size and decorations
3. Visual requirements—good visual acuity or corrected through glasses
4. Instructions can be given verbally, written, or through demonstration

SUPPLIES

- 4-inch clay pot and base
- Scrap wallpaper or wrapping paper with designs that can be cut out
- Decoupage
- Paint brush
- Scissors
- Three colors of acrylic paint
- Small, rounded sponge

PRECAUTIONS

Hot glue can burn fingers. Clients will need to be proficient in using a glue gun or the gluing can be done for them. Clients with painful joints may find pulling apart flower stems, wrapping ribbon, and making bows difficult or uncomfortable to complete. Children will need to have glueing done for them.

ACTIVITY GRADATION

Client can follow predetermined pattern for wreath, or design own for more creativity. Gluing can be done for the client. Size of wreaths can vary greatly.

NOTE Wreaths can be made from dried or silk flowers. They can have a seasonal theme or can be used year round. Other materials could include spiced apples, cinnamon sticks, and spices (i.e., bay leaves). Let your personal taste show through in your choice of colors and materials.

Client Information for Wreath Making

SUPPLIES

- 4-inch clay pot and base
- Scrap wallpaper or wrapping paper with designs that can be cut out
- Decoupage
- Paint brush
- Scissors
- Three colors of acrylic paint
- Small, rounded sponge

INSTRUCTIONS

1. Select dried or silk flowers and greenery to be used in your project.

   Note: Needle nose pliers are helpful to pull silk flowers apart because of wires in them.

2. Choose wreath.
3. On the wreath, decide where center point of the bottom half is to be for later placement of the bow (Figure 11-1).
4. Wrap wreath with ribbon, starting at center point and glue to the wreath at start and finish points.

Figure 11-1

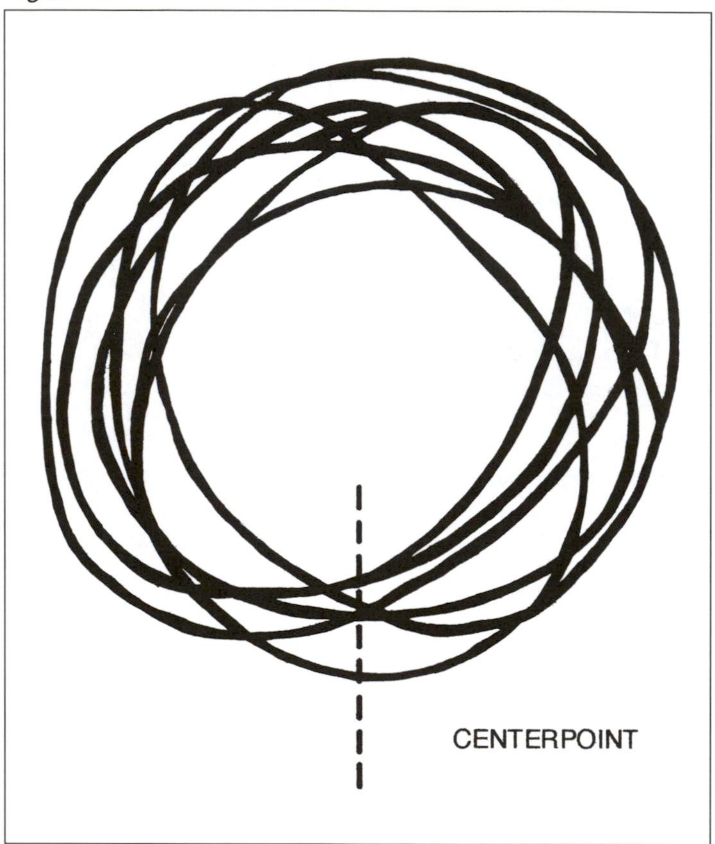

5. Arrange longer stems, probably greenery, and glue to wreath and start and finish points.
6. Add shorter stems, fanning out from center point again.
7. Make a 6-inch loop bow with long tails using wire in center to keep bow from unraveling.
8. Glue bow to center point (Figure 11-1).
9. Fill in spaces with smaller stems or flowers such as baby's breath or German statice.

   Note: Web-like glue strands may form when gluing with a glue gun. Wait until wreath is completed and dried, then remove simply by gently pulling them off.

CORRECTING MISTAKES

Stems can gently be pulled off and re-glued if necessary.

CARE OF PROJECT

Dust carefully by gently shaking wreath or blowing on it.

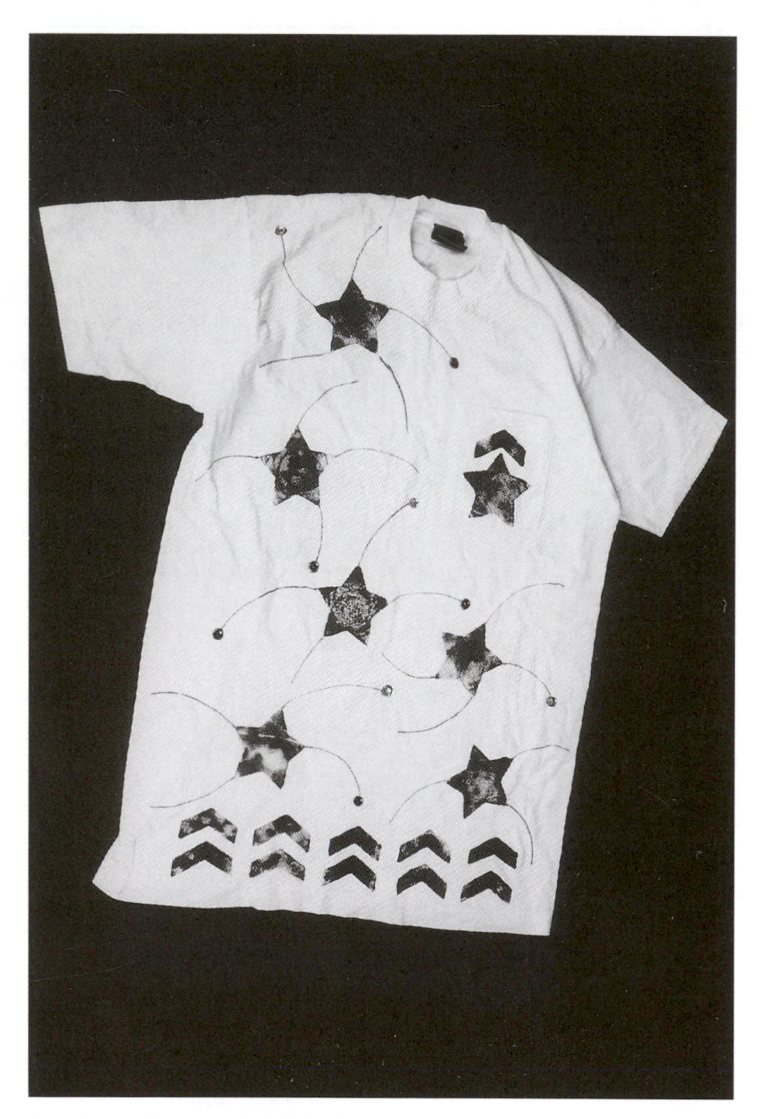

Sponge-Stamped T-shirt

Chapter 12

SPONGE-STAMPED T-SHIRT

Therapist Information for Sponge-Stamped T-shirt

ACTIVITY ANALYSIS

Clients can turn ordinary T-shirts into a work of art. Stamping can be done with pre-cut sponge shapes or can be cut out of regular sponges for individual preferences and designs. This project is quickly completed, including drying time. It can be done in steps and several sessions if the design is more complex. This is a cognitive/perceptual task that requires use of gross motor coordination.

This project may enhance performance in the following component areas:

Motor Components

- Fine motor abilities of the hand
- Coordination of the hand/arm
- Hand dominance
- Endurance

Cognitive Components

- Organizational abilities
- Problem-solving abilities
- Ability to plan
- Concentration
- Attention to task
- Sequencing ability
- Decision-making skills

Perceptual Components

- Eye-hand coordination
- Awareness of spatial relations
- Tactile awareness in the hands
- Motor planning of hands and upper extremities

Emotional Components

- Self-esteem

Social Components

- Ability to work alone

Adaptations

- Position required—sitting upright or standing
- Can be unilateral with use of adaptive equipment
- High success rate
- Can vary from a structured to an unstructured activity
- Can be done individually
- Can be adapted for a group
- Design could incorporate some individual culture values

GENERAL INFORMATION

1. Age—child through adult
2. Cost—minimal to moderate
3. Visual requirements—could be completed with mild visual deficits
4. Instructions can be given verbally, written, or through demonstration

SUPPLIES

- T-shirt
- Blue fabric paint
- Red fabric paint
- Gold fabric paint
- Plastic or paper plate
- Fabric rhinestones (not sew-on variety)
- Large piece of cardboard

PRECAUTIONS

- Should not be used with clients who have PICA behaviors (those who eat non-food items).
- Some respiratory clients may be affected by paint smell, although minimal on this project.
- Check labels on paint for toxicity.

ACTIVITY GRADATION

Project can be done in predetermined design. Project can use pre-cut sponges to simplify task, or client may cut his or her own sponge for hand strengthening.

Project can allow for creativity in design, color, and other embellishments (i.e., rhinestones, bows, buttons). You can use an old T-shirt and make it new or use an undecorated new T-shirt. This project will take only a little time to complete and after drying overnight can be worn. Follow our design or make up one of your own. Cut sponges into any shape to create an original shirt.

NOTE

Client Information for Sponge-Stamped T-shirt

SUPPLIES

- T-shirt
- Blue fabric paint
- Red fabric paint
- Gold fabric paint
- Plastic or paper plate
- Fabric rhinestones (not sew-on variety)
- Large piece of cardboard

INSTRUCTIONS

1. Wash and dry T-shirt.
2. Put piece of cardboard inside T-shirt from seam to seam to fill up all of the shirt.
3. Squirt desired color of paint onto a plate.
4. With sponge, spread and pat paint, to even out paint on the plate, and coat bottom surface of the sponge evenly.
5. When sponge surface is covered with paint, place on T-shirt and press down firmly and evenly, being careful not to move the sponge.
6. Lift the sponge gently and evenly, trying not to smear paint design.
7. Repeat steps 5 and 6 with second color and a different sponge.

8. With gold paint tube, add lines or outline shapes, squeezing right from the tube onto the shirt.
9. To add rhinestones, squirt gold paint in one place until the same size as the rhinestone.
10. Gently place rhinestone on top of paint drop.
11. Gently push down until paint surrounds the rhinestone.
12. Allow paint to dry overnight.

CORRECTING MISTAKES

It is difficult to remove any smudged or misplaced paint. However, additional designs or rhinestones could be added to hide these mistakes.

CARE OF PROJECT

Turn shirt inside out before washing. Wash on gentle cycle in cold water and line dry.

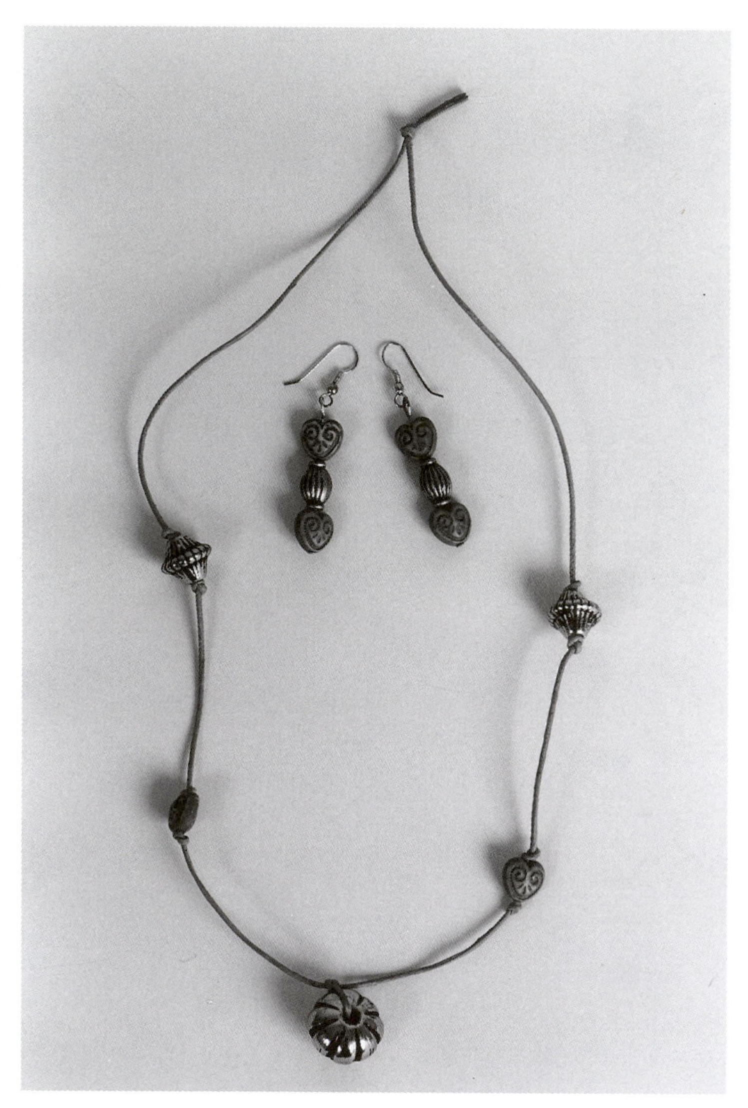

Jewelry

Chapter 13

JEWELRY

Therapist Information for Jewelry

ACTIVITY ANALYSIS

This costume jewelry craft is inexpensive as it does not use precious metals; it can be completed in a minimal amount of treatment time. Clients can use creativity in the selection of materials, beads, colors, and combinations thereof. This is an especially good craft for increasing self-esteem. It could become a vocational task if the client becomes proficient at the process. This activity is a bilateral activity with emphasis on fine motor skills.

This project may enhance performance in the following component areas:

Motor Components

- Fine motor abilities of the hand
- Use of hands bilaterally
- Strength

Cognitive Components

- Organizational abilities
- Problem-solving abilities
- Ability to plan
- Concentration
- Attention to task
- Sequencing ability
- Decision-making skills

Perceptual Components

- Eye-hand coordination
- Awareness of spatial relations
- Tactile awareness in the hands
- Constructional apraxia

Emotional Components

- Independence
- Self-esteem
- Self expression

Social Components

- Ability to work alone

Adaptations

- Position required—sitting upright or reclining in bed
- Allows for repetition of hand and finger motions
- High success rate
- Can vary from a structured to an unstructured activity
- Can be done individually

GENERAL INFORMATION

1. Age—child through adult
2. Cost—minimal
3. Visual requirements—necklace could be done by tactility; however, the earrings require good visual acuity
4. Instructions can be given verbally, written, or through demonstration

SUPPLIES

- Package of head pins
- Package of fish hook ear wires
- Package of desired beads
- Fine leather lacing
- Needle nose pliers
- Scissors

PRECAUTIONS

Precautions with sharp objects are necessary when using scissors, and precautions with patients with PICA behaviors (those who eat non-food items) should be observed.

ACTIVITY GRADATIONS

Beads and pattern could be chosen for client. You may increase or decrease the number of beads used.

NOTE This project can be done quickly and provide you with accessories that will "make" your outfit. These jewelry pieces have become popular items at craft bazaars. The choice of colors and types of beads can express your individuality. The choices are unlimited.

Client Information for Jewelry

SUPPLIES

- Package of head pins
- Package of fish hook ear wires
- Package of desired beads
- Fine leather lacing
- Needle nose pliers
- Scissors

INSTRUCTIONS

Earrings

1. String beads onto head pin in desired order.
2. Using needle nose pliers, bend head pin end to a right angle.
3. Make a loop in the opposite direction using the pliers (Figure 13-1).
4. Include loop of ear wire before closing head pin loop tightly.

   Note: If head pin is too long for amount of beads chosen, use pliers to bend excess back and forth until it breaks off. Make sure to leave enough to make the loop.

Necklace

1. Measure desired length of fine leather lace (18 inch).
2. Choose middle bead, preferably a larger bead.
3. Slide large bead onto fine leather lace until at middle.

Figure 13-1

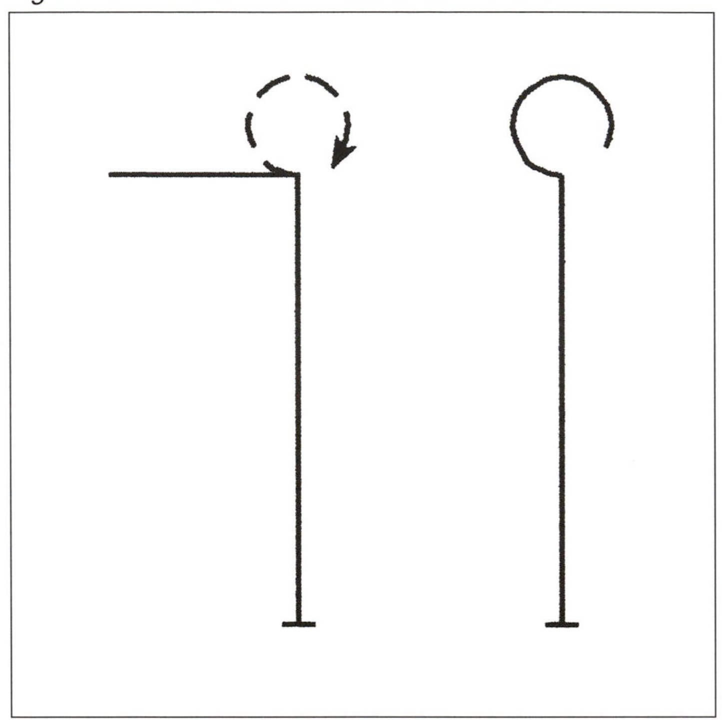

4. Tie a knot of either side of large bead
5. On each lace, tie a knot approximately 2 inches from the large bead.
6. Add bead or beads as desired and tie knot again in each lace to hold beads in place.
7. Add as many knots and beads as desired.
8. Tie two lace ends together in knot to finish.

CORRECTING MISTAKES

Slide beads off lacing and untie knots if changes are needed.

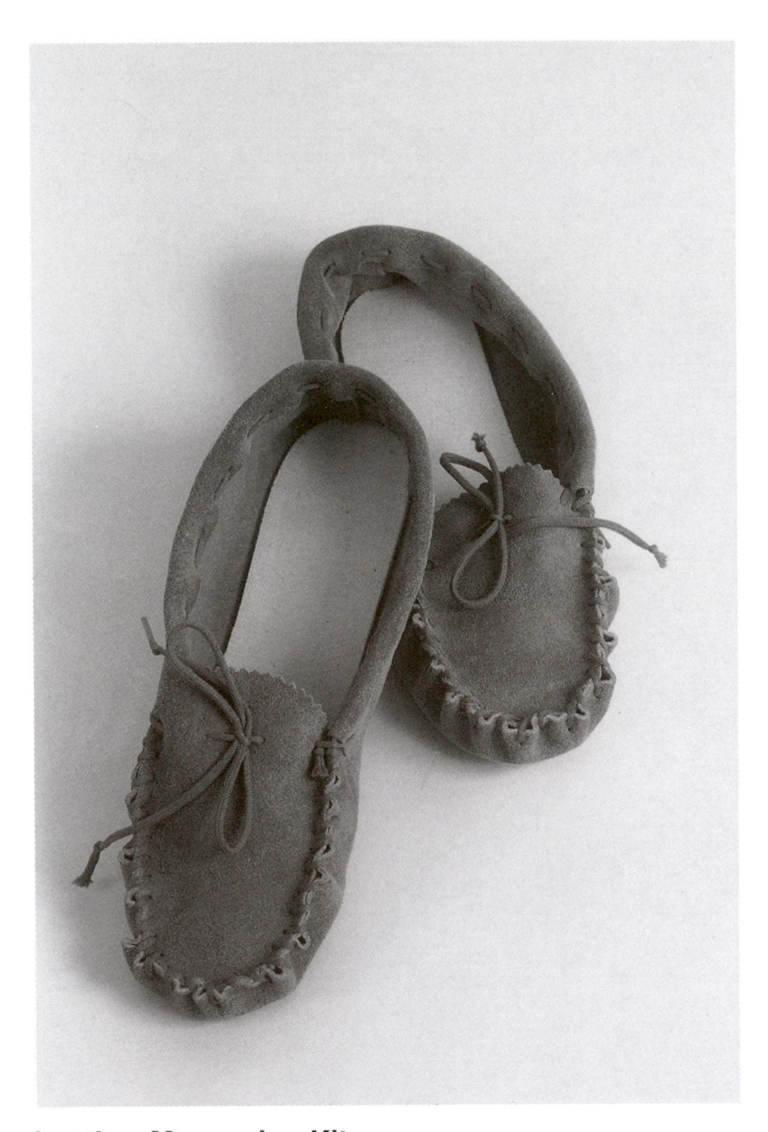

Leather Moccasins Kit

Chapter 14

LEATHER MOCCASINS KIT

Therapist Information for Leather Moccasins Kit

ACTIVITY ANALYSIS

This leather moccasin kit is a fine product from the S&S Arts and Crafts Catalog. The leather pieces are precut and prepunched with holes for lacing. The assembly process is relatively simple, so the finished project is satisfying and useful for the client. This is a highly successful project. This craft emphasizes precision prehension, fine motor strengthening with gross motor components.

This project may enhance performance in the following component areas:

Motor Components

- Fine motor abilities of the hand
- Coordination of the hand/arm
- Use of hands bilaterally
- Endurance
- Strength

Cognitive Components

- Problem-solving abilities
- Concentration
- Sequencing ability

Perceptual Components

- Eye-hand coordination
- Tactile awareness in the hands
- Motor planning of hands and upper extremities
- Constructional apraxia

Emotional Components

- Independence
- Self-esteem

Social Components

- Ability to work alone

Adaptations

- Position required—sitting upright or reclining in bed
- Allows for repetition of hand and finger motions
- High success rate
- Can be done individually
- Design could incorporate some individual cultural values

GENERAL INFORMATION

1. Age—adolescence to adult
2. Cost—moderately priced kit
3. Visual requirements—fair visual acuity, as good sense of touch can compensate
4. Instructions can be given verbally, written, or through demonstration

SUPPLIES

- S&S Arts and Crafts Catalog kit number LE-528M (1-800-243-9232)
- Needle nose pliers
- A large nail
- Scissors

PRECAUTIONS

Generally a safe task. However, scissors are needed to trim lacing and should be used with care. This craft may be contraindicated for clients with carpal tunnel syndrome and involvement of the small joints of the hand.

ACTIVITY GRADATION

This kit does not readily lend itself to gradation.

NOTE Here is a craft you can wear when you are done. The S&S Leather Moccasin Kit provides you with everything you need to complete a pair of comfortable leather moccasins. This project increases your strength and fine coordination.

Client Information for Leather Moccasins Kit

SUPPLIES

- S&S Arts and Crafts Catalog kit number LE-528M (1-800-243-9232)
- Needle nose pliers
- A large nail
- Scissors

INSTRUCTIONS

1. Tie a simple knot in one end of a lace.
2. From the outside of the "vamp" (or sole of the moccasin) draw lace through holes of vamp and "plug" (piece that covers your toe). In the first hole, draw the lace through twice to make a secure beginning (Figure 14-1).
3. Use a large nail and place it between plug and vamp (Figure 14-2). Make the next stitch and draw it tight.
4. Lace all around the toe using the nail between the plug and vamp at each stitch. Pull each stitch tight for an even look.

   Note: The edge of the vamp should look puckered between stitches.
5. Go through last hole twice to securely fasten both pieces (Figure 14-3).
6. Tie a knot loosely at the lace and work it down so the knot is close to the hole to eliminate any slack lacing (Figure 14-4).
7. Cut off surplus lacing and save it for the heel.
8. Next fold the square ends of the heel and tie at the top temporarily.
9. Knot the piece of lace left from the toe and lace it through the heel (Figure 14-5).
10. Finish off with another knot.
11. Fold the cuff and put it in place.
12. Take another lace and draw it through the holes of the plug and vamp (Figure 14-6).

13. Leave at least 7 inches of the lace at the toe end.
14. Lace all around the cuff, going in and out (Figure 14-7).
15. Pass the end of the lace in and out of the two plug holes and put the moccasin on your foot.
16. Draw lace tight to a comfortable fit and tie a bow.
17. Repeat all above steps for completion of the second moccasin.

CORRECTING MISTAKES

Pull lacing out and straighten and start again. Note: Needle nose pliers can make it easier to pull the lacing through the holes. If plastic lace ends come off, wrap end with tape.

Figure 14-1

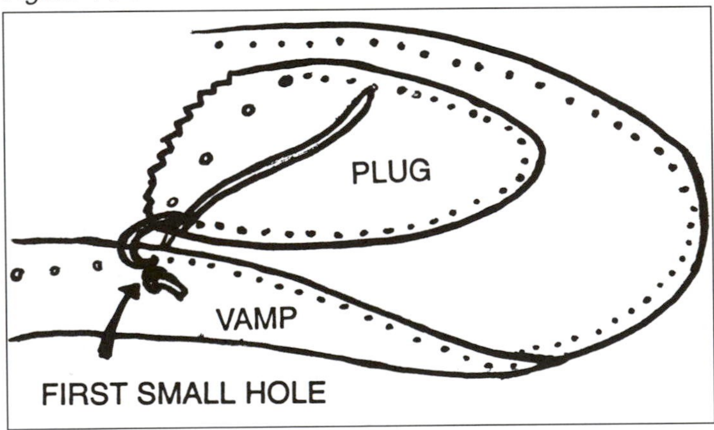

Figure 14-2

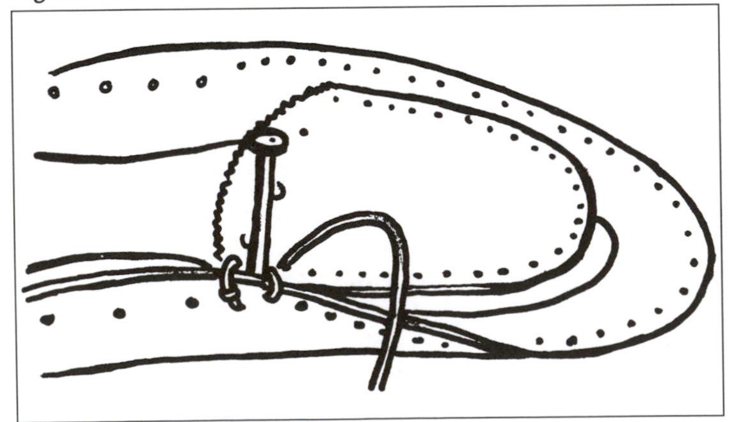

Figure 14-3

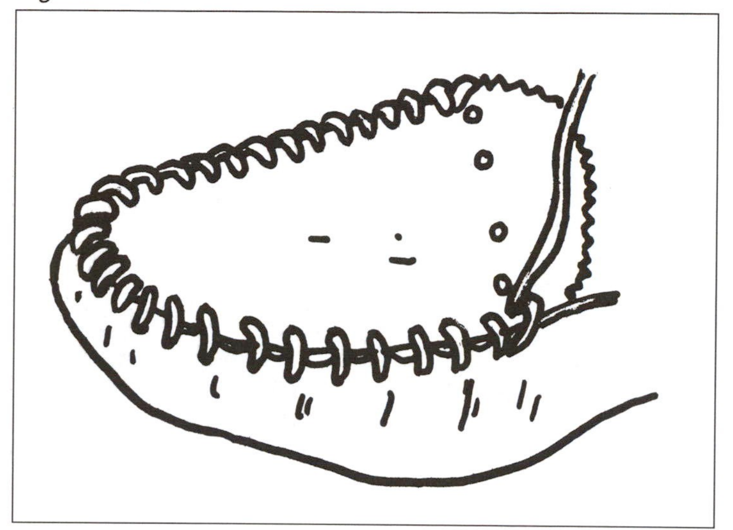

Figure 14-4

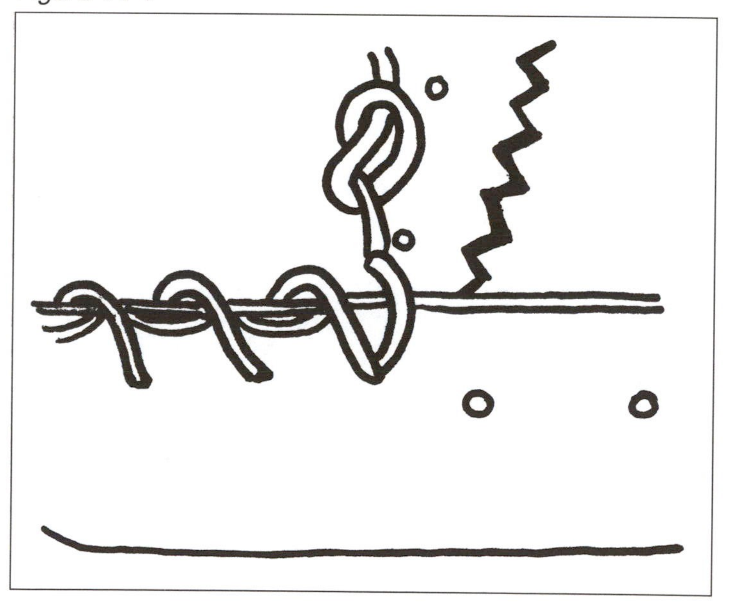

Figure 14-5

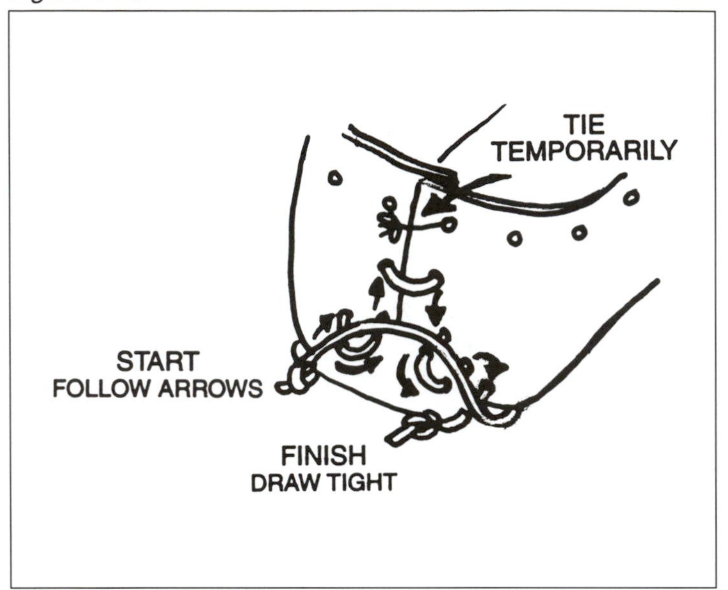

Figure 14-6

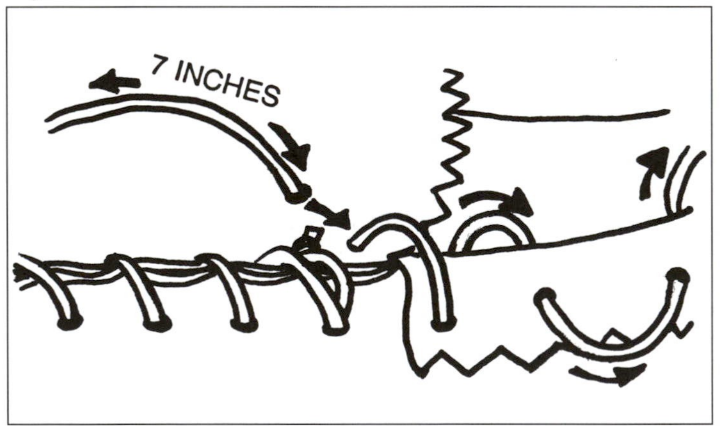

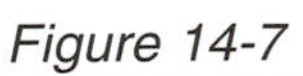

Figure 14-7

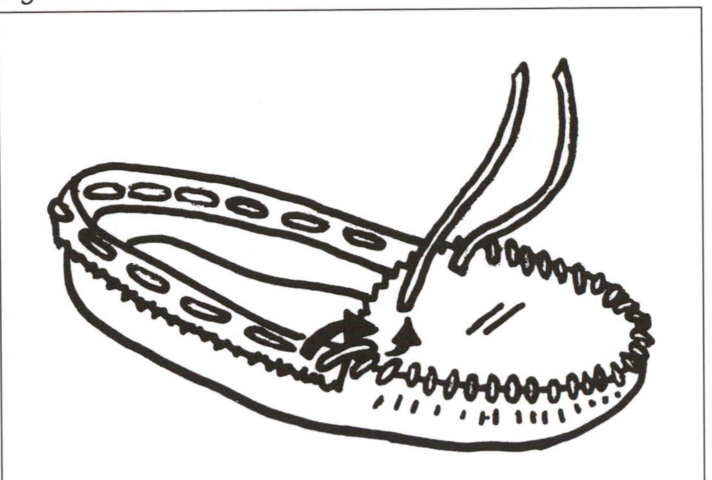

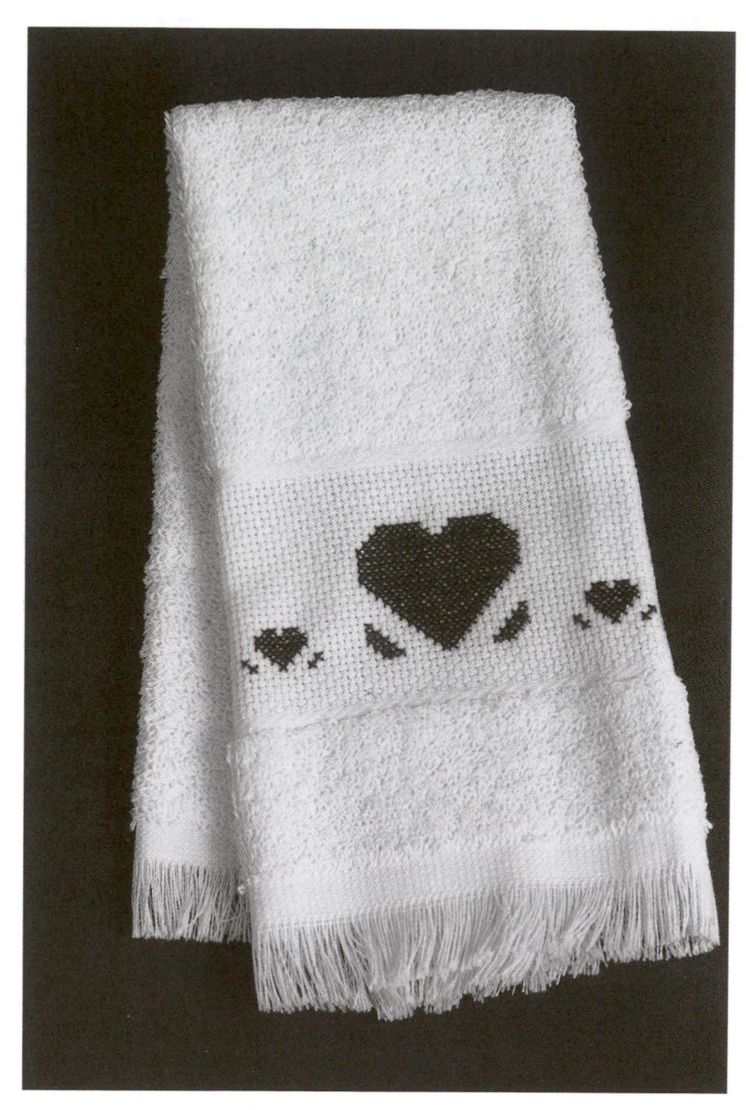

Counted Cross-Stitch Towel

Chapter 15

COUNTED CROSS-STITCH TOWEL

Therapist Information for Counted Cross-Stitch Towel

ACTIVITY ANALYSIS

Cross-stitch has become a very popular form of stitchery, perhaps because of how even and perfect the results can be. Stitching is done on evenly woven fabrics such as Aida Cloth and designs can be chosen from multitudes of books, magazines, and leaflets. Clients can create their own designs on graph paper. Designs are available for the novice or the expert stitcher. This cognitive task emphasizes fine motor skills. It is a good craft to consider for changing dominance or one-handed training with adaptive equipment.

This project may enhance performance in the following component areas:

Motor Components

- Fine motor abilities of the hand
- Coordination of the hand/arm
- Hand dominance
- Endurance

Cognitive Components

- Organizational abilities
- Concentration
- Attention to task
- Sequencing ability
- Decision-making skills

Perceptual Components

- Eye-hand coordination
- Awareness of spatial relations
- Motor planning of hands and upper extremities

Emotional Components

- Independence
- Self-esteem

Social Components

- Ability to work alone

Adaptations

- Position required—sitting upright or reclining in bed
- Allows for repetition of hand and finger motions
- Can be used for one-handed training, with use of adaptive equipment
- High success rate
- Can be done individually
- Design could incorporate some cultural values of an individual

GENERAL INFORMATION

1. Age—teenager through adult
2. Cost—inexpensive to moderate, depending on the fabric chosen
3. Visual requirements—good visual acuity or corrected with glasses
4. Instructions can be given verbally, written, or through demonstration

SUPPLIES

- Scissors
- Blunt tip needle
- Six-strand embroidery floss (our sample used red and green)
- Cross-stitch hand towel

PRECAUTIONS

Precautions with sharp objects are necessary when using scissors and needle. May be difficult for those with tremors or severe incoordination, and may be contraindicated for clients with carpal tunnel syndrome or involvement of the small joints of the hand.

ACTIVITY GRADATION

This project can be varied depending on design and size of cloth used. This project can be the beginning of a leisure craft that will provide hours of enjoyment.

NOTE Cross-stitch can be very relaxing and satisfying. The stitch is very simple to learn and beyond that, you only need to know how to count.

Client Information for Counted Cross-Stitch Towel

SUPPLIES

- Scissors
- Blunt tip needle
- Six-strand embroidery floss (our sample used red and green)
- Cross-stitch hand towel

INSTRUCTIONS

1. Cut embroidery floss into 18-inch lengths.
2. Separate the six strands into three parts. You will use only two strands when making the design.
3. Thread the needle with two strands of red floss. Do not knot the threads.
4. Find the center of the design on the graph marked by the arrows.
5. Find the center of the towel by folding it in half lengthwise.
6. From the bottom center of the towel, count up four squares. Move over one square to the left. The first stitch will be on the bottom of the large heart on the pattern grid included.

   Note: When starting the first stitch, hold the end of the thread loosely on the back side of the fabric and secure with first couple of stitches.
7. Mark one cross stitch for each "x" and "o" on the pattern.

   Note: The "x" and the "o" represent different colors (Figure 15-1).
8. Work all horizontal rows across in one direction and then work back (Figure 15-2).
9. Work the next rows up the fabric until the design is completed.
10. To secure finish at the end, weave the floss through the back of several stitches.

Figure 15-1

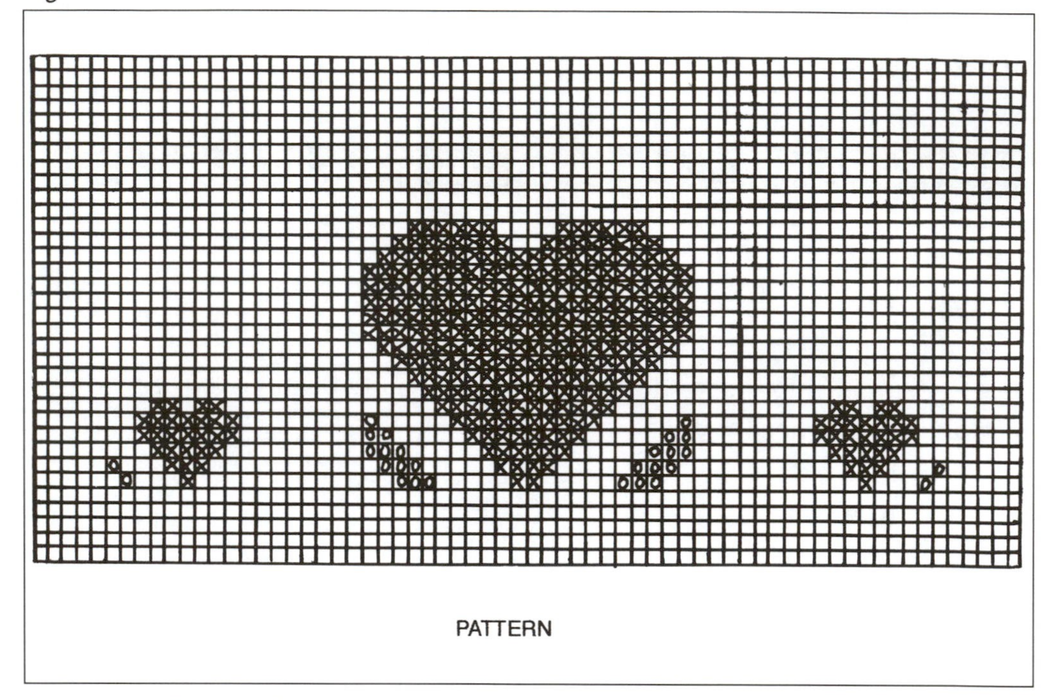

PATTERN

Figure 15-2

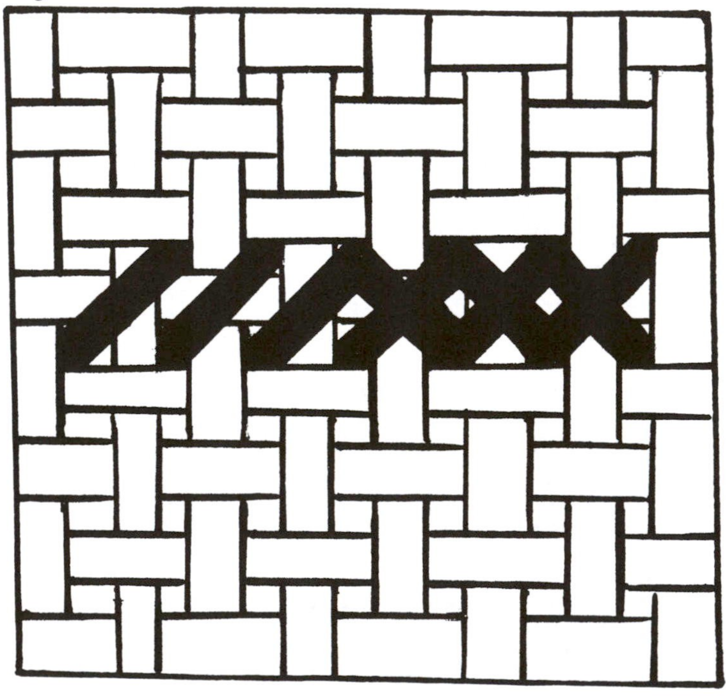

11. Cut off excess floss.
12. Start stitching second color, counting spaces between, as shown on the graph.

CARE OF PROJECT

The project can be machine washed on gentle cycle, in cold water, and dried in the dryer.

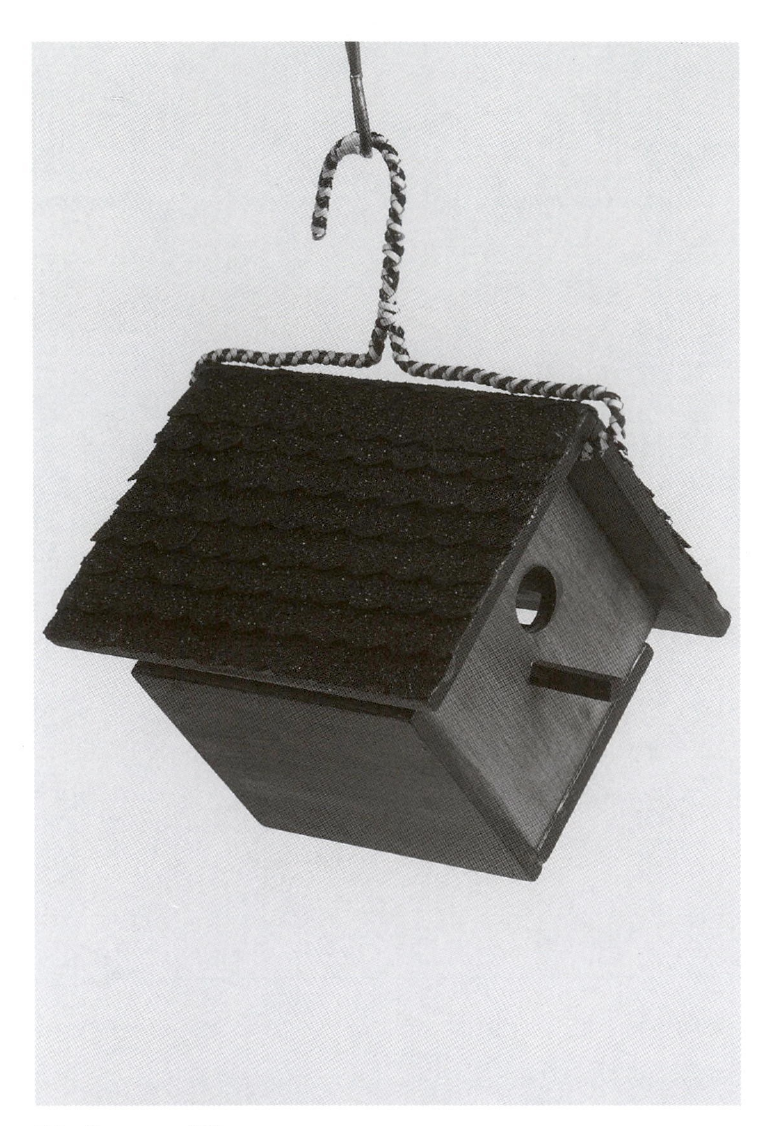

Birdhouse Kit

Chapter 16

BIRDHOUSE KIT

Therapist Information for Birdhouse Kit

ACTIVITY ANALYSIS

The birdhouse kit is a fine product from the S&S Arts and Crafts Catalog. The pieces are precut of soft pine and can be sanded easily. The assembly process is relatively simple so that the finished project is satisfying for the client to complete. The birdhouse can be individualized by using acrylic paints instead of stains. As with our sample, shingles can be added to the roof and various types of hangers can be added to secure the birdhouse to the tree. There is a high success rate with this project. This is a gross motor task, good for strengthening upper extremity muscle groups. May be helpful in changing hand dominance or in one-handed training.

This project may enhance performance in the following component areas:

Motor Components

- Fine motor abilities of the hand
- Coordination of the hand/arm
- Hand dominance
- Use of hands bilaterally
- Endurance
- Strength

Cognitive Components

- Problem-solving abilities
- Ability to plan
- Attention to task
- Sequencing ability
- Decision-making skills

Perceptual Components

- Eye-hand coordination

- Awareness of spatial relations
- Tactile awareness in the hands
- Motor planning of hands and upper extremities
- Constructional praxia

Emotional Components

- Independence
- Self-esteem
- Release of negative feelings

Social Components

- Comfort level in group settings
- Ability to work alone

Adaptations

- Position required—sitting upright or standing
- Allows for repetition of hand and finger motions
- Can vary from a structured to an unstructured activity
- Can be done individually

GENERAL INFORMATION

1. Age—teenage through adult.
2. Cost—S&S Arts and Crafts Catalog Birdhouse Kit No. WD-602 is minimal in cost, plus the cost for paint or varnish
3. Visual requirements—good visual acuity or corrected with glasses
4. Instructions can be given verbally, written, or through demonstration

SUPPLIES

- S&S Arts and Crafts Catalog, Kit No. WD-602 (1-800-243-9232). Kit contains
  one square front with hole
  one square back
  two smaller rectangular pieces for sides
  two larger rectangular pieces for roof
  wooden perch
  sandpaper
  nails
- Acrylic paint or stain of choice
- Paint brushes or foam rubber brush

- Carpenter's glue
- White glue
- Soft cloths
- Hammer or small awl

PRECAUTIONS

Precautions should be observed with small awl. Contraindicated for clients with pulmonary conditions, due to sawdust and varnish.

ACTIVITY GRADATION

Tape wood pieces to table to keep in place when sanding. It could be assembled without sanding or staining for a respiratory client. Adding shingles and braided hanger can increase level of complexity. Attach such things as birch bark and doll house parts (wood cutouts and shapes) to individualize the project. Could be sanded on an incline board for upper extremity strengthening with or without use of weights.

NOTE Making a birdhouse can satisfy your creative energies as well as strengthening your shoulder and elbow muscles. The birdhouse kit contains all the pieces you need to complete the task, a functional home for your feathered friends.

Client Information for Birdhouse Kit

SUPPLIES

- S&S Arts and Crafts Catalog, Kit No. WD-602 (1-800-243-9232). Kit contains
  one square front with hole
  one square back
  two smaller rectangular pieces for sides
  two larger rectangular pieces for roof
  wooden perch
  sandpaper
  nails
- Acrylic paint or stain of choice
- Paint brushes or foam rubber brush
- Carpenter's glue
- White glue

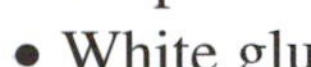

- Soft cloths
- Hammer or small awl

INSTRUCTIONS

1. Sand all wood pieces until very smooth, especially edges.
2. Wipe off all dust with soft cloth.
3. Stain or paint wood pieces to desired color scheme. Let pieces dry 30 minutes. Sample birdhouse is stained with walnut stain.

Putting on the Perch

1. Take square front piece with hole in it and from the back side, drive a nail toward the front so that the tip of the nail is coming through. Place nail about ½ inch below hole.
2. Put glue on end of perch piece and put glued end over nail tip and set aside for a few minutes so the glue can harden a bit.
3. Rest perch on the table and pound the nail into the perch to secure it to the birdhouse front.
4. Pound nail in gently.

Forming the Birdhouse Walls

1. Determine which surface of the smaller rectangular pieces will be the outside of the birdhouse. One of the two pieces is slightly larger than the other.
2. Into the larger piece, make three starter holes evenly spaced with a small awl and bring the longer side about ¼ inch in from the edge.
3. Put three nails into the starter holes and pound them through the wood so just the tip of the nail shows through on the back side.
4. Take the smaller of these side pieces and put glue along one of the longer edges.
5. Place the nail tips from the larger piece over the glue and pound the nails into both pieces to form a "V." This will be the bottom of the birdhouse (Figure 16-1).

Putting on the Front and Back

1. Place one half of the "V" on the table and let the other half hang over the edge.
2. Make two pilot holes on each end to attach the front and back pieces to the sides of the birdhouse (Figure 16-2).
3. Drive the nails through the wood so the tips of the nails show through other side.
4. Turn the "V" around and put nails in the other side also.
5. Put the back square piece into the "V" and nail the side pieces to the back.
6. Put the front piece, with perch, into the other side of the "V" and nail in place.

   Note: Be sure to nail the perch side on the outside.

Figure 16-1

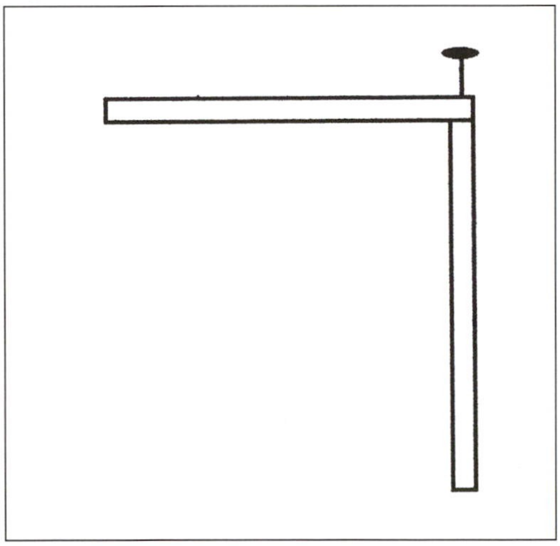

Making the Roof

1. Determine which surface of the larger rectangular pieces will be the outside of the birdhouse. One of the pieces is slightly larger than the other.
2. Into the larger piece, make three starter holes evenly spaced with a small awl along the longer side about ¼ inch in from the edge.

Figure 16-2

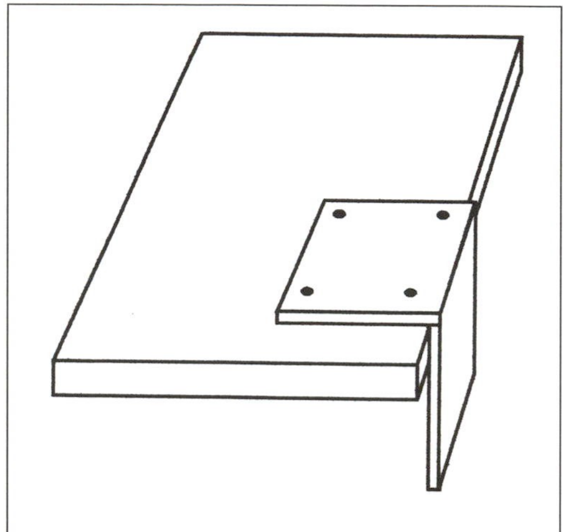

3. Put four nail holes and pound them through the wood so just the tips of the nails show through on the back side.
4. Take the smaller of these roof pieces and put glue along one of the longer edges.
5. Place the nail tips from the larger piece over the glue and pound the nails into both pieces to form a "V" (Figure 16-1).

Placing the Roof on the Birdhouse

This is tricky because you have to determine where the nails go by touch and an exact measurement. If the nails are off, you will not secure the roof to the body of the birdhouse.

1. Center the roof piece over the birdhouse.
2. Nail the roof to the front and back pieces. You may wish to reinforce the bond by putting glue on the two edges of the front and back pieces before nailing it in place.

   Note: There is approximately an inch of air space showing between the roof and the sides of the birdhouse. This is supposed to be there so the birds do not overheat in the birdhouse.

Our sample has had an asphalt roof added for trim. The shingle material was purchased at a local doll house supplier. The hanger was made from a clothes hanger. The larger hook is easier to attach to tree branches. We braided leather lacing over the hanger for additional decoration.

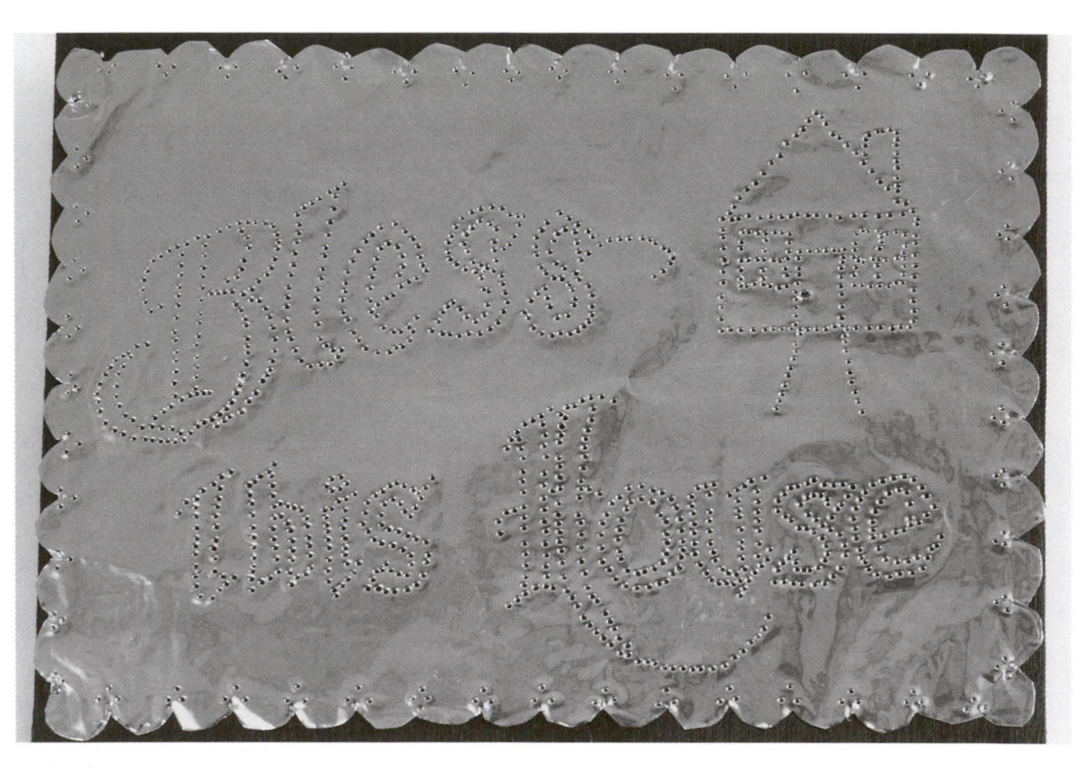

Nail Art

Chapter 17

NAIL ART

Therapist Information for Nail Art

ACTIVITY ANALYSIS

Nail art is an excellent activity for strengthening a shoulder, for bilateral use of the hands, and, strangely enough, for changing dominance (with the assistance of the therapist) and also for working on visual field neglect. It is also a project that involves familiar tools, so that it would be a good task for men or women who don't like to do crafts. The finished project is very pleasing and can be mounted on a wood plaque very easily.

This project may enhance performance in the following component areas:

Motor Components

- Fine motor abilities of the hand
- Coordination of the hand/arm
- Hand dominance
- Use of the hands bilaterally
- Endurance
- Strength

Cognitive Components

- Organizational abilities
- Problem-solving abilities
- Ability to plan
- Concentration
- Attention to task

Perceptual Components

- Eye-hand coordination
- Awareness of spatial relations
- Tactile awareness in the hands
- Motor planning of hands and upper extremities

Emotional Components

- Independence
- Self-esteem
- Release of negative feelings

Social Components

- Ability to work alone

Adaptations

- Position required—sitting upright or standing
- Allows for repetition of hand and finger motions
- Can be used for one-handed training, with therapist's help to hold the awl
- High success rate
- Can be done individually
- Design could incorporate some individual cultural values

GENERAL INFORMATION

1. Age—teenager through adulthood
2. Cost—moderate
3. Visual requirements—good visual acuity and ability to look into visual field neglect
4. Instructions can be given verbally, written, or through demonstration

SUPPLIES

- Metal foil (copper, gold colored, or aluminum)
- Small awl or large nail
- Hammer, can be graded light to heavy
- Magazines or wooden backboard
- Wood board on which to mount metal foil

PRECAUTIONS

Precautions should be observed when using a small awl. The hammer could be used as a weapon by an agitated or a psychotic client. Edges of the metal foil should be covered by masking tape to prevent cuts to client and infection control precautions should be observed if puncture or bruising are a concern for a client. This activity may be stressful to small joints of the hands.

ACTIVITY GRADATION

Therapist can hold the awl (with his or her hand or a pair of pliers depending upon the skills of the client) and the client can use the hammer only (for unilateral use by client or to help change dominance).

The hammer can range from a tack hammer to a 3-pound construction hammer. Weights can be added to the client's upper extremities for improving strength. There are more steps if copper foil is used because of the finishing steps. The design can be simple or more complex, with more or less holes.

NOTE Using a nail to make a picture may sound like a strange thing to do, but the results are quite striking. The project will help strengthen muscles as well as satisfy aesthetic senses. The design is made by placing a nail or small awl tip on the dots in the pattern and transferring the pattern to metal foil. This project will make a fine gift for a friend or relative.

Client Information for Nail Art

SUPPLIES

- Metal foil (copper, gold colored, or aluminum)
- Small awl or large nail
- Hammer, can be graded light to heavy
- Magazines or wooden backboard
- Wood board on which to mount metal foil

INSTRUCTIONS

1. Cut a piece of metal foil 8½ inches by 12 inches.
2. Wrap the edge of the metal foil with masking tape to prevent cuts.
3. Center the pattern on the metal foil piece.
4. Put metal foil and pattern on several magazines or a piece of metal scrap wood to protect table surface.
5. Place the small awl tip onto the dots in the pattern and hit with a hammer to puncture foil.
6. Continue until all dots on the pattern have been punctured and whole design has been transferred (Figure 17-1).

Figure 17-1

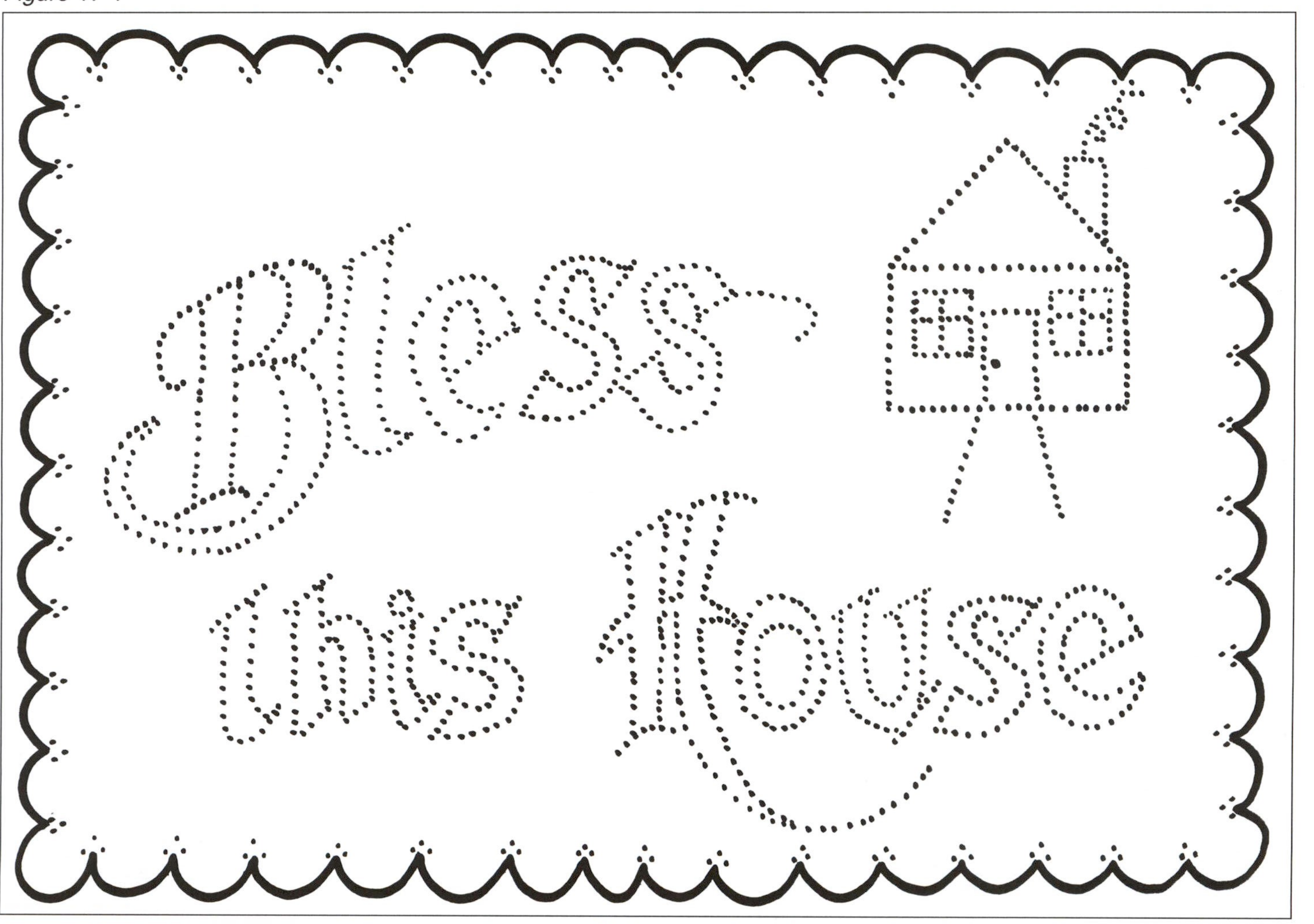

7. To check to see if you have missed any dots/holes, turn the foil pattern over and compare with the pattern.
8. To finish off the design, take an orange stick with a blunt tip and draw the curved lines in the frame. Push hard to make a deep impression.

To Mount Metal Foil Picture

1. Cut a wooden board 9 inches by 12½ inches.
2. Sand board smooth, especially on the edges.
3. Paint the board black so that the nail holes show better.
4. Using small escheon pins, nail the metal foil design to the board.

Optional

You could carefully cut the metal foil around the scallop design to give your picture a custom finish. Be careful not to cut your fingertips on the metal edges.

CORRECTING MISTAKES

Once a hole has been made in the metal foil it cannot be removed.

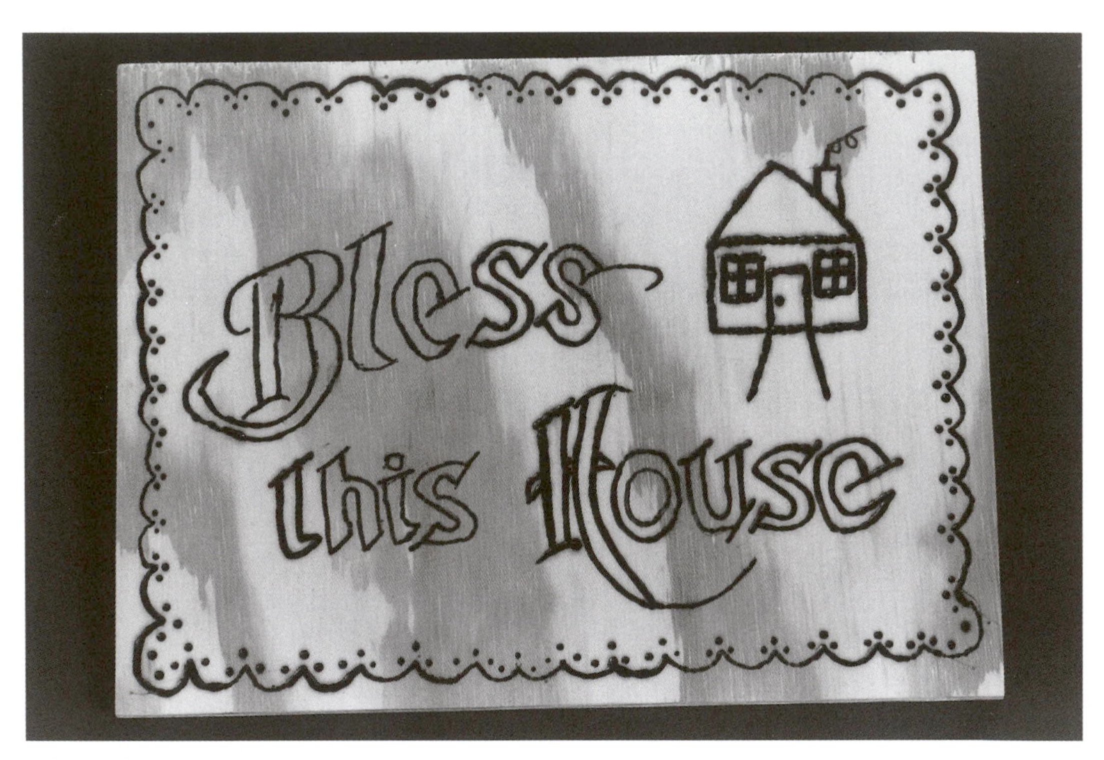

Wood Burning

Chapter 18

WOOD BURNING

Therapist Information for Wood Burning

ACTIVITY ANALYSIS

Woodburning is an ancient craft. It has an added benefit of providing some olfactory stimulation as well as muscle strengthening and coordination. The finished project is pleasing to look at and can be designed to use a multitude of shading for very dramatic effects. It has an element of danger because of the hot tool used so it can be a preliminary evaluation for safety and judgment before use of more sophisticated power tools. This is a good task for changing hand dominance, by doing the whole design with the non-dominant hand.

This project may enhance performance in the following component areas:

Motor Components

- Fine motor abilities of the hand
- Coordination of the hand/arm
- Hand dominance
- Hand strength

Cognitive Components

- Organizational abilities
- Problem-solving abilities
- Ability to plan
- Concentration
- Attention to task

Perceptual Components

- Eye-hand coordination
- Awareness of spatial relations
- Motor planning of hands and upper extremities

Emotional Components

- Independence
- Self-esteem

Social Components

- Ability to work alone

Adaptations

- Position required—sitting upright at a table
- Allows for repetition of hand and finger motions
- Can be unilateral with use of adaptive equipment
- Can be done individually
- Design could incorporate some individual cultural values

GENERAL INFORMATION

1. Age—teenager through adult
2. Cost—once you have wood burning tool and a small supply of wood pieces, the task is relatively inexpensive
3. Visual requirements—good visual acuity or corrected with glasses
4. Instructions can be given verbally, written, or through demonstration

SUPPLIES

- Wood piece ½ inch bigger than the pattern
- Graphite paper
- Pattern
- Pencil
- Woodburning tools with various tips
- Holder for woodburning tool
  Soft cloth
- Varnish or finishing oil
- Sandpaper

PRECAUTIONS

The woodburning tool is hot. It must be in a holder or on an asbestos pad when not in use. Hold tool on handle only. Do not touch end to see if it is hot enough. Instead, try burning a few strokes on a piece of scrap wood. Do not use with impulsive clients. Smell of burning wood may be a problem for clients with respiratory disease. May not be appropriate for clients with severe visual neglect.

ACTIVITY GRADATION

By making the pattern larger or with more detail, you can increase the complexity of the project. By offering the client choice of tips to use to enhance the shading of the finished project, the complexity of the task increases.

NOTE Wood burning can be a very satisfying activity. It can produce a picture or design that is relatively simple, but by shading different areas, it can look very complicated. Wood burning requires a person to pay close attention to the work being done; however, it can be started and stopped easily. This technique works well for making signs that could be hung outdoors as the design will not wash off in bad weather. Wood burning can also be used to make very delicate designs. It is a versatile craft.

Client Information for Wood Burning

SUPPLIES

- Wood piece ½ inch bigger than the pattern
- Graphite paper
- Pattern
- Pencil
- Woodburning tools with various tips
- Holder for woodburning tool
- Soft cloth
- Varnish or finishing oil
- Sandpaper

INSTRUCTIONS

1. Select desired pattern, one without a lot of fine detail (Figure 18-1).
2. Cut a piece of wood large enough to accommodate the pattern.

   Note: Avoid using plywood as it distorts the effect of the "burning."
3. Sand the face of the wood so that it is very smooth. The edges can be sanded now or later.
4. Place a piece of graphite paper face down on the wood.
5. Place the pattern over the graphite paper and tape in place.

Figure 18-1

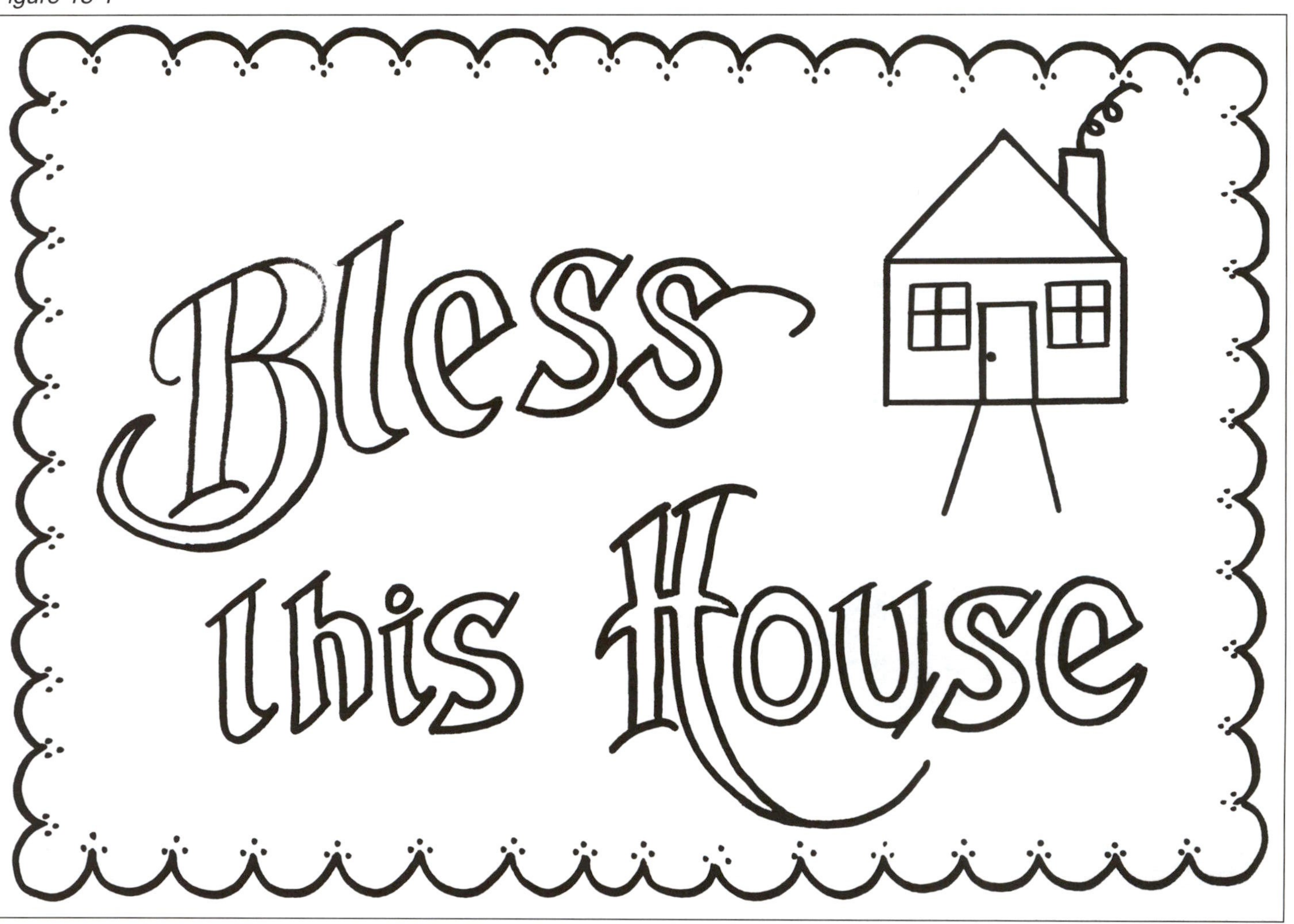

6. Trace over the pattern to transfer the pattern to the wood.
7. Remove the pattern and the graphite paper.
8. Plug in and heat the wood burning tool.

   Note: Be sure the tool rests on a holder to keep it off the table or place it on an asbestos pad for safety.
9. Practice using the wood burning tool on a piece of scrap wood.

   Note: a) Make random marks until you feel comfortable with the tool, b) do not hold the wood burning tool in one space too long as it will make unwanted scorch marks. Keep fingers away from the tool's hot end.
10. Start burning over the traced pattern on the wood.
11. Wood burn the whole design onto the wood board.
12. Sand the edges of the board if not already done.
13. Varnish or apply finishing oil to the surface of the design to preserve the wood. Our sample project was oiled with linseed oil.
14. Add hanger to reverse side of the board.

CORRECTING MISTAKES

If it is not too deep, the mistake can be lightly sanded out. The mistake could be incorporated into the design by shading.

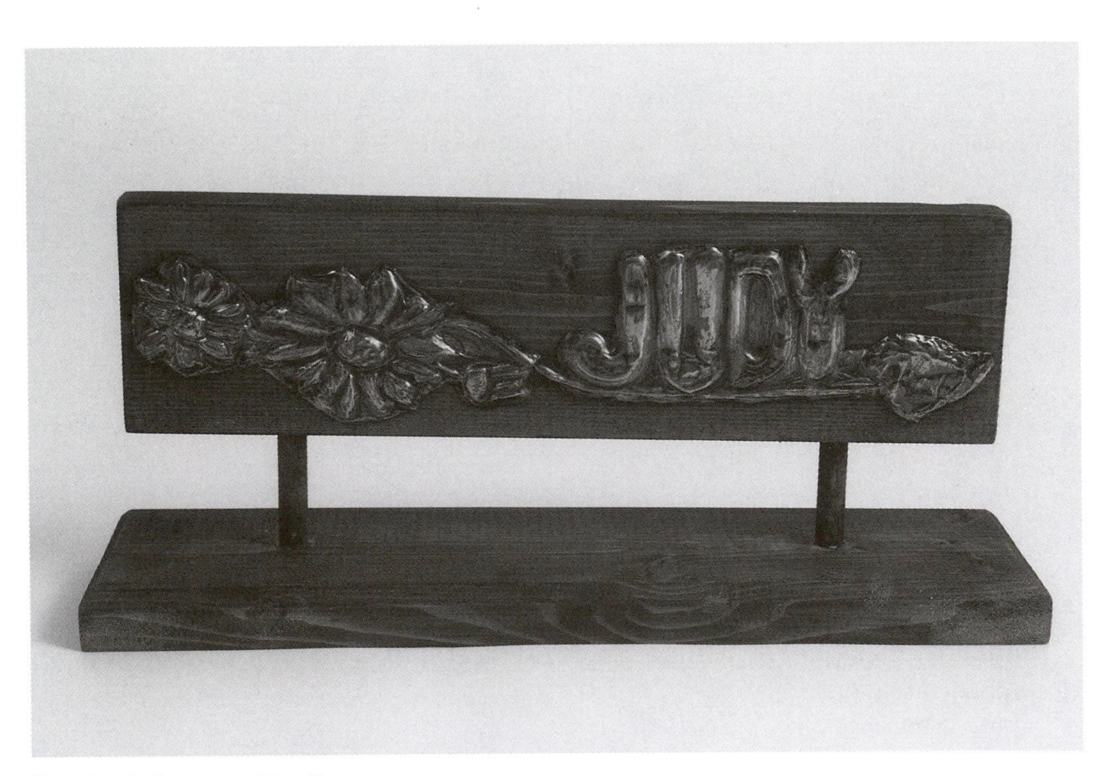

Original Copper Tooling

Chapter 19

ORIGINAL COPPER TOOLING

Therapist Information for Original Copper Tooling

ACTIVITY ANALYSIS

Copper tooling is a fascinating technique that requires patience and determination. Results can be very elegant. Once the metal piece is antiqued, the highlights especially enhance the design. Copper tooling can be customized very easily so the client's own designs or name can be used. Designs used in copper tooling need to be simple. This is not a medium for detail work. This craft can be bilateral or unilateral depending on set up. This is a high level cognitive task, requiring the ability to mentally manipulate information in order to complete the task.

This project may enhance performance in the following component areas:

Motor Components

- Fine motor abilities of the hand
- Coordination of the hand/arm
- Hand dominance
- Strength

Cognitive Components

- Organizational abilities
- Problem-solving abilities
- Ability to plan
- Concentration
- Attention to task
- Sequencing ability

Perceptual Components

- Eye-hand coordination
- Awareness of spatial relations
- Tactile awareness in the hands

- Motor planning of the hands and upper extremities

Emotional Components

- Independence
- Self-esteem

Social Components

- Ability to work alone

Adaptations

- Position required—sitting upright at a table
- Allows for repetition of hand and finger motions
- Can be unilateral with use of adaptive equipment
- Can be done individually
- Design could incorporate some cultural values of an individual

GENERAL INFORMATION

1. Age—teenager through adult
2. Cost—minimal
3. Visual requirements—good visual acuity or corrected with glasses
4. Instructions can be given verbally, written, or through demonstration. In this task, demonstration is often helpful

SUPPLIES

- Copper foil sheets, ½ inch larger than design
- Pattern
- Graphite paper
- Orange sticks of various sizes, ½ inch down to pencil point in diameter
- Magazines or newspaper for work surface
- Wood board to mount project
- Liver of sulphur
- Cotton tipped swabs to apply liver of sulphur
- Steel wool
- Silicone spray to seal copper, once finished
- Modeling clay

PRECAUTIONS

The metal piece is worked from both sides so the edge of the metal foil needs to be covered with masking tape to protect the client from cuts. The chemicals used to antique the copper are toxic and need to be closely supervised. This task would require static positioning and downward force to the small joints of the hands.

ACTIVITY GRADATION

This is a complex, multi-step task. It would be difficult to simplify it, unless portions are done by the therapist.

NOTE Making original copper tooling designs can express a person's individuality. No one else will have a design exactly like yours. The metal is worked from both sides and the design is initially put onto the metal backwards. That is so the finished project will have the design "pushed out front."

Client Information for Original Copper Tooling

SUPPLIES

- Copper foil sheets, ½ inch larger than design
- Pattern
- Graphite paper
- Orange sticks of various sizes, ½ inch down to pencil point in diameter
- Magazines or newspaper for work surface
- Wood board to mount project
- Liver of sulphur
- Cotton tipped swabs to apply liver of sulphur
- Steel wool
- Silicone spray to seal copper, once finished
- Modeling clay

INSTRUCTIONS

1. Cut a piece of copper foil 3 inches by 12 inches.
2. Tape the edges of the copper foil with masking tape to prevent cuts.
3. Print your name in the dotted box in the pattern (Figure 19-1).

4. Tape graphite paper to the back of the pattern (with the graphite toward the back of the pattern page).
5. Trace over the pattern to transfer the design to the back side of the pattern sheet.
6. Turn the pattern over and remove the graphite paper.
7. Use this reverse pattern to transfer the design to the copper foil.
8. Tape the reverse pattern to the copper foil so it will not shift.
9. Put metal foil on magazine or newspaper pad.
10. Use a dull pencil or dull-tipped orange stick to transfer the design to the copper foil.
11. Trace over the whole design to transfer it to the copper foil.
12. Take the pattern off the metal foil.
13. Turn the metal foil over.
14. Use the pointed end of an orange stick and press around the outer edge of the design as close as possible.
15. Use a ½-inch diameter orange stick to flatten areas surrounding the design.
16. Turn over the metal piece to the back and push out the design with the flat edge of a pencil-size orange stick.

    Note: This makes the design prominent on the front side of the metal foil.
17. Fill the back side of the design with modeling clay for support.
18. Use steel wool lightly on the front side of the project to get off all oily fingerprints.
19. Wipe with a clean, dry cloth.
20. Put three drops of liver of sulphur into approximately 2 ounces of water and mix with a cotton swab.
21. Apply mixture to front of design to antique the finish. It is okay if it turns black.

Figure 19-1

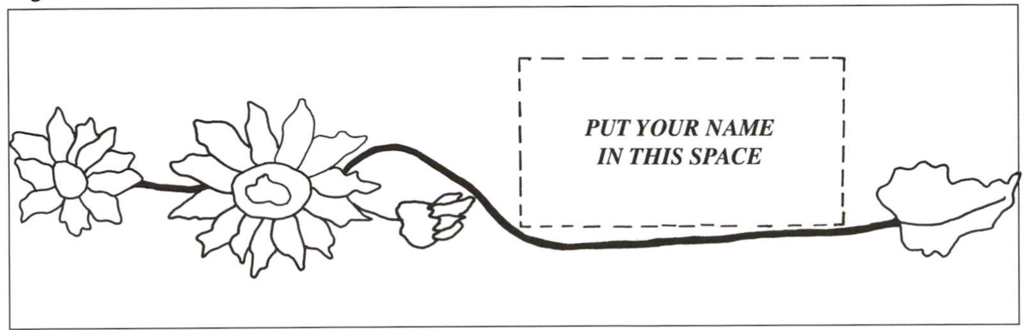

22. Rub steel wool on the surface of the front of the design to give luster and bring out the highlights on the copper.

    Note: Polish depending on how much of the highlights you want developed.

23. Spray the project with silicone spray to maintain the luster.
24. Trim off the excess copper. In our sample we cut to the design. You could leave it a rectangle if you prefer.
25. Mount project to wooden board with copper escheon pins.

CORRECTING MISTAKES

Work the copper from either side to sharpen the design. Work the copper gently or it will rip, then it cannot be repaired. You would have to start over.

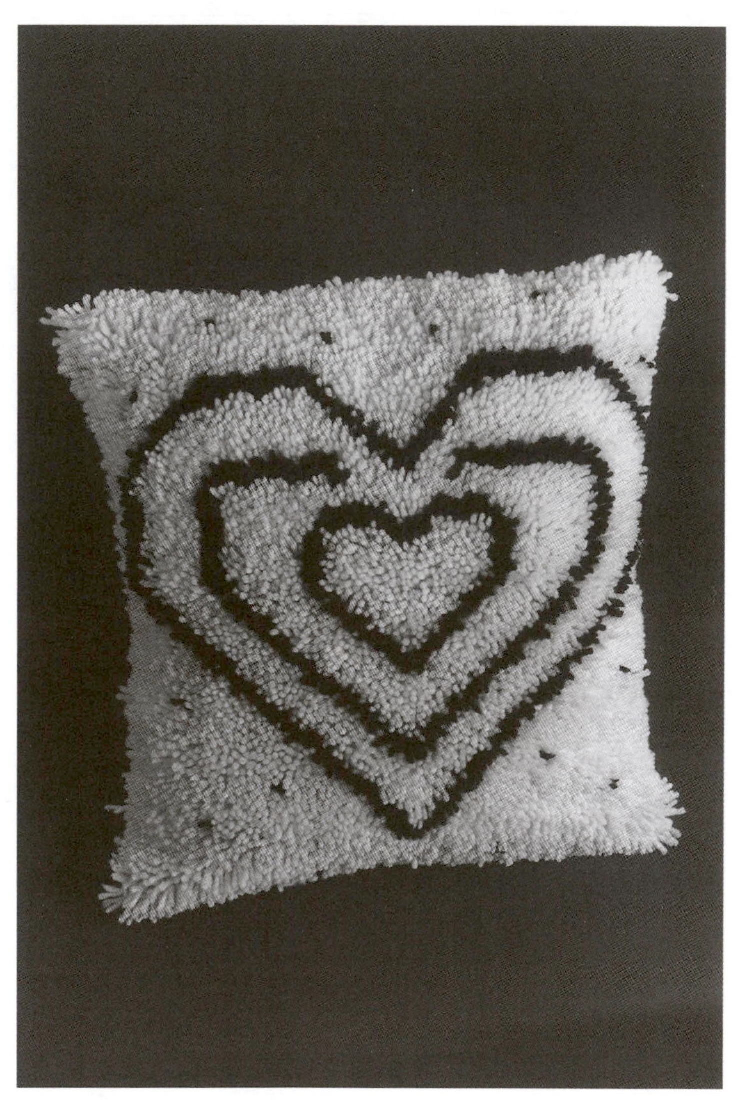

Latch Hook

Chapter 20

LATCH HOOK

Therapist Information for Latch Hook

ACTIVITY ANALYSIS

Once you get the rhythm of latch hooking, this activity can be very restful. Designs can vary from easy to complex. With this craft, it is easy to design your own pattern. Many things can be made from latch hook, including wall hangings, pillows, and rugs. Latch hook is considered a long-term project taking many hours to complete. This is a bilateral task using fine motor skills to hold yarn pieces and gross motor skills to manipulate the latch hook. There is strong visual/perceptual components to this task.

This project may enhance performance in the following component areas:

Motor Components

- Fine motor abilities of the hand
- Coordination of the hand/arm
- Use of hands bilaterally
- Endurance
- Strength

Cognitive Components

- Organizational abilities
- Ability to plan
- Concentration

Perceptual Components

- Eye-hand coordination
- Awareness of spatial relations
- Tactile awareness in the hands
- Awareness of the neglected side

Emotional Components

- Independence
- Self-esteem

Social Components

- Ability to work alone

Adaptations

- Position required—reclining or sitting upright
- Allows for repetition of hand and finger motions
- High success rate
- Can be done individually
- Design could incorporate some cultural values of an individual

GENERAL INFORMATION

1. Age—teenager to adult
2. Cost—moderate
3. Visual requirement—good visual acuity or corrected with glasses
4. Instructions can be given verbally, written, or through demonstration

SUPPLIES

- Latch hook canvas
- Latch hook
- Pieces of yarn cut into 2 1/2-inch lengths
- Colors: natural (6 bags), pink (4 bags), red (2 bags)
- Each bag contains 320 pieces
- Masking tape
- Scissors

PRECAUTIONS

Precautions with sharp objects are necessary when using scissors. If a patient is on suicide precautions, he or she should not be given a whole ball of yarn to cut into pieces unless closely supervised. If task is worked for an extended period of time, rotator cuff muscles or carpal tunnel syndrome may be aggravated.

ACTIVITY GRADATION

Canvas can be left blank if following the pattern as with counted cross stitches procedures. An individual's pattern can be marked onto blank canvas to make it easier to follow. A kit containing all materials and a preprinted canvas can be used for maximal structure for the client.

NOTE Latch hook can provide hours of relaxation. It can be worked in front of the television, in an easy chair, or while waiting at the doctor's office, for example. You can create your own pattern on a blank canvas or use a preprinted canvas in a kit. The finished project will provide you with much satisfaction. The sample shown in this book can be used as a pillow.

Client Information for Latch Hook

SUPPLIES

- Latch hook canvas
- Latch hook
- Pieces of yarn cut into 2 1/2-inch lengths
- Colors: natural (6 bags), pink (4 bags), red (2 bags) (Figure 20-1)
- Each bag contains 320 pieces
- Masking tape
- Scissors

INSTRUCTIONS

1. Put masking tape around the edges of the canvas to protect your skin during work.
2. Begin at the bottom of the work. Always hook in one direction, left to right, or right to left, whichever is more comfortable.
3. Fold one piece of yarn around latch hook shaft, leaving latch hook open (Figure 20-2a).
4. Insert latch hook into hole of canvas mesh and up through the hole directly above it (Figure 20-2b).
5. Twist yarn ends into the space under the C shape of the hook. The latch will close as the hook is pulled back out of the canvas (Figure 20-2c).
6. Pull the hook quickly to make the knot form.

Figure 20-1

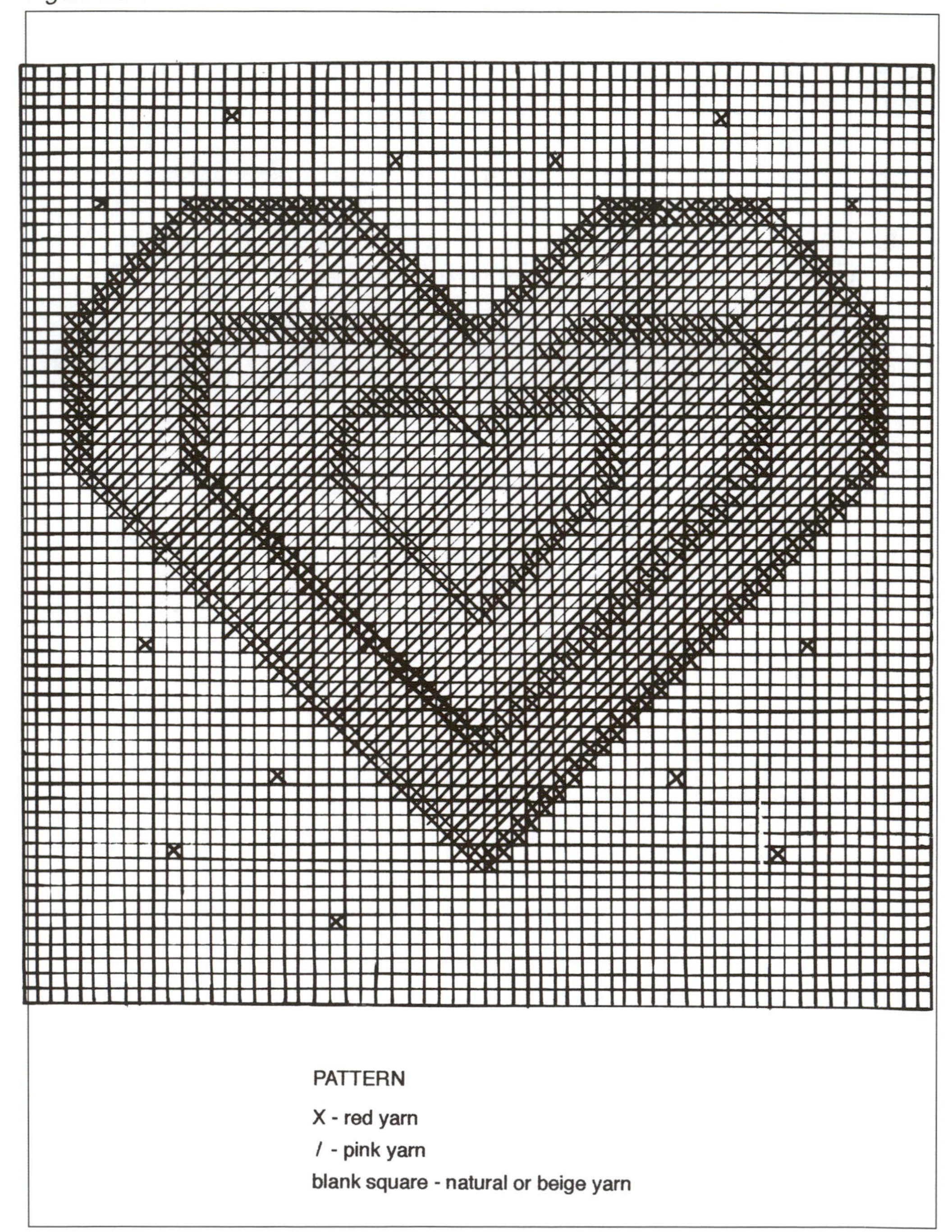

PATTERN

X - red yarn

/ - pink yarn

blank square - natural or beige yarn

7. Tug ends of the yarn to tighten knot.
8. Repeat steps 3 through 7 until done.

   Note: Clip any uneven yarn pieces to even out the pile.

CORRECTING MISTAKES

Pull out incorrect pieces of yarn and work pattern again.

CARE OF PROJECT

Wet or dry shampoo can be used on this project by following the directions on commercially available products.

Figure 20-2

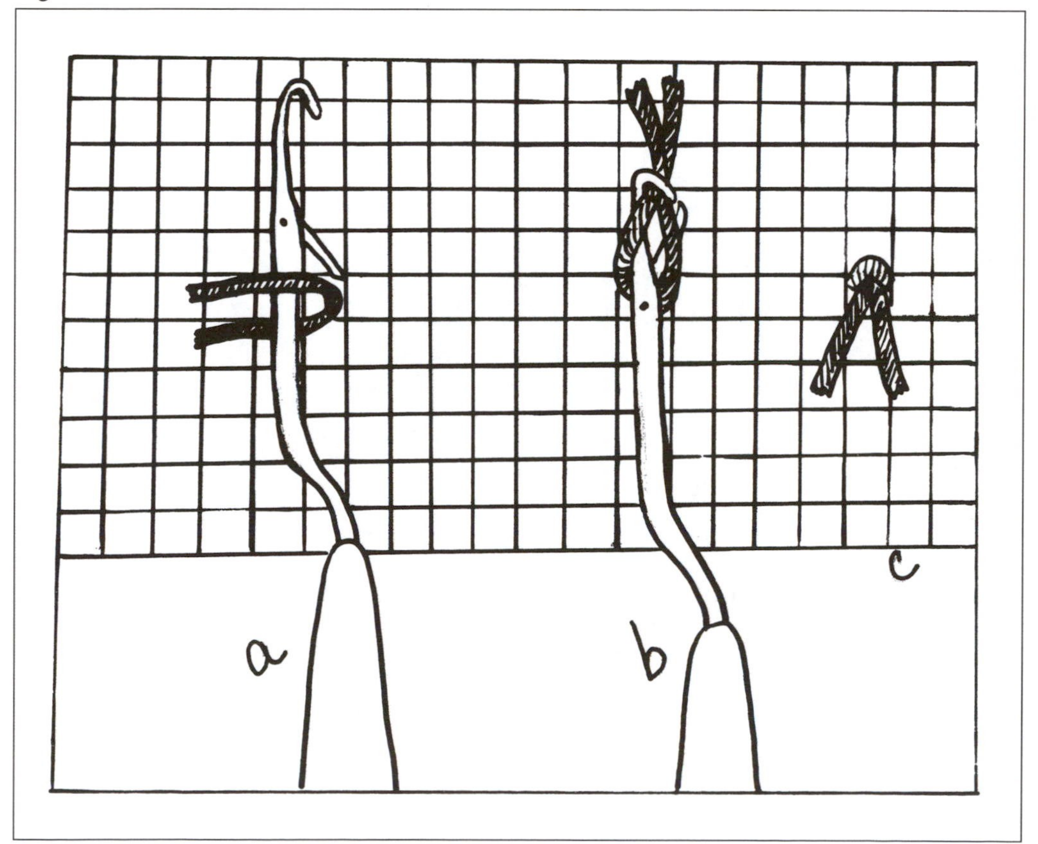

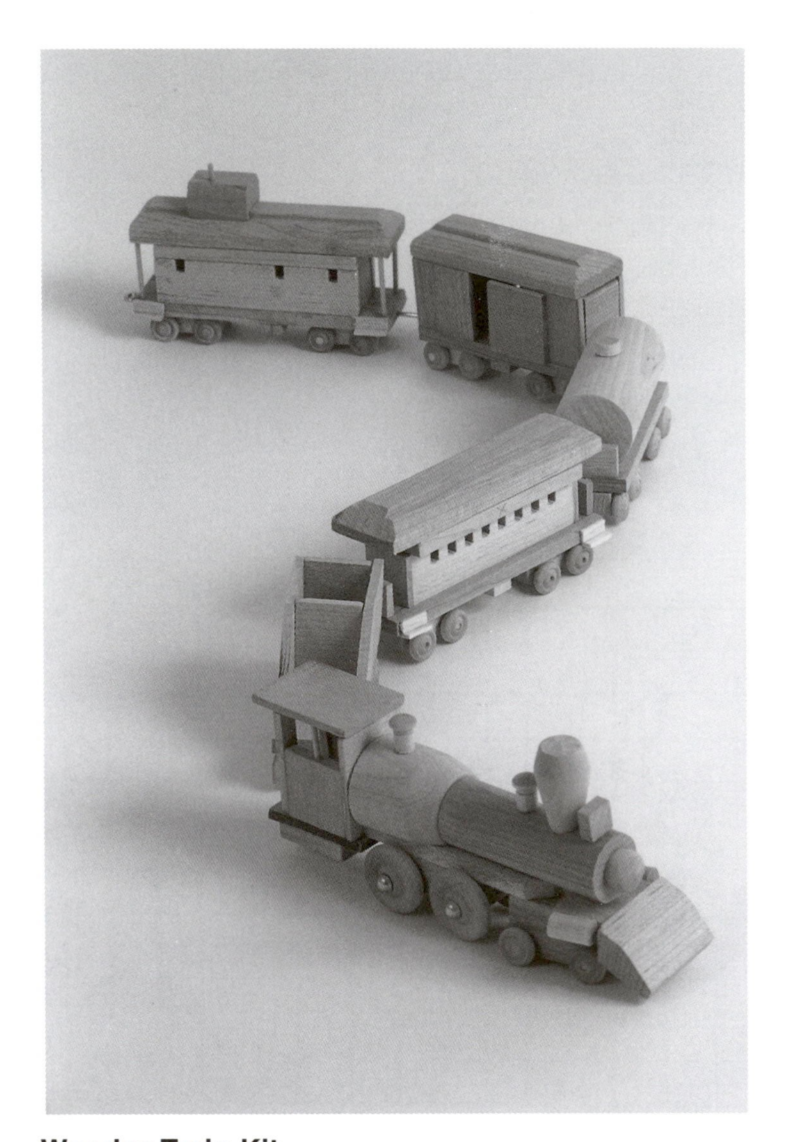

Wooden Train Kit

Chapter 21

WOODEN TRAIN KIT

Therapist Information for Wooden Train Kit

ACTIVITY ANALYSIS

Kits are convenient to use. Everything you need is included in the kit and preparation is minimal. The step-by-step instructions are included with the kit. This wooden train kit from S&S Arts and Crafts Catalog is challenging. Because of the small parts, it takes planning and is good for working on organizational skills. It is also a good task to use for developing independent working skills that include increasing problem-solving skills. This task requires good fine motor skills and good visual acuity.

This project may enhance performance in the following component areas:

Motor Components

- Fine motor abilities of the hand
- Coordination of the hand/arm
- Use of the hands bilaterally
- Endurance

Cognitive Components

- Organizational abilities
- Problem-solving abilities
- Ability to plan
- Concentration
- Attention to task
- Sequencing ability
- Decision-making skills

Perceptual Components

- Eye-hand coordination
- Awareness of spatial relations
- Tactile awareness in the hands

- Motor planning of the hands and upper extremities
- Constructional praxia

Emotional Components

- Independence
- Self-esteem

Social Components

- Sociability in new situations
- Ability to work alone

Adaptations

- Position required—sitting upright or reclining
- Allows for repetition of hand and finger motions
- High success rate
- Can be done individually
- Can be adapted for a group

GENERAL INFORMATION

1. Age—8 years to adult
2. Cost—expensive, but broken down by number of clinic treatments, it is reasonable
3. Visual requirements—good visual acuity or corrected with glasses
4. Instructions can be given verbally or written. The project can be assembled by looking at the picture along with only a few verbal clues for clarification

SUPPLIES

- Train kit No. GA 2297 from S&S Arts and Crafts Catalog (1-800-243-9232)
- Glue
- Cotton swabs for applying the glue
- Sandpaper
- Ruler
- Pencil
- Needle nose pliers
- Acrylic paints, varnish, or finishing oil (optional)

PRECAUTIONS

Close supervision is needed for younger children because of small pieces that could be swallowed. Not to be used with a client who has PICA behaviors (those who eat non-food items). May be difficult for those clients with tremors, severe incoordination, or small hand joint pain.

ACTIVITY GRADATION

The project can be made more difficult by increasing the decoration of the train cars, by adding decals, or by making the wheels movable versus static.

NOTE This task provides the challenge of taking small pieces and assembling them into an attractive decoration for the home or a toy for a child. It looks authentic and can be decorated with color or left in natural wood tones.

Client Information for Wooden Train Kit

SUPPLIES

- Train kit No. GA 2297 from S&S Arts and Crafts Catalog (1-800-243-9232)
- Glue
- Cotton swabs for applying the glue
- Sandpaper
- Ruler
- Pencil
- Needle nose pliers
- Acrylic paints, varnish, or finishing oil (optional)

INSTRUCTIONS

1. Written instructions are provided with each car of the train kit. Review them.

   Note: It is helpful to mark the pieces lightly with a pencil on one side so they will not be confused during assembly. Make your own system to identify the pieces such as marking them A, B, or C on what will become the inside of the train surface.

2. Sand pieces as necessary for a smooth finish.
3. Have a plate with a small pile of glue. Use the cotton swab to apply glue to small pieces.
4. If you want the wheels on the train cars to be movable, you need to sand the entire length of the dowel slightly to allow movement in the hole. Excessive sanding, however, will make the wheels fall off.

CORRECTING MISTAKES

You will need to correct any mistakes quickly. Once the glue has dried, errors are almost impossible to correct.

CARE OF PROJECT

It can be dusted or wiped off with a damp cloth. Do not immerse in water.

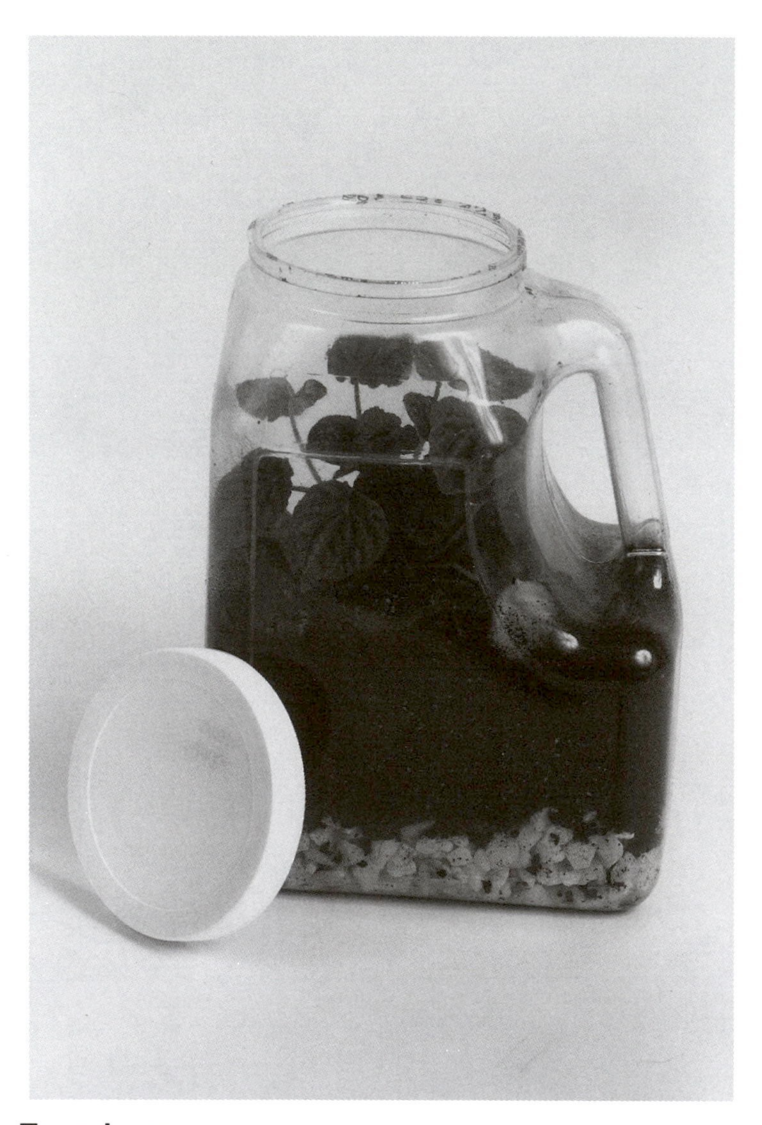

Terrariums

Chapter 22

TERRARIUMS

Therapist Information for Terrariums

ACTIVITY ANALYSIS

This is an attractive craft involving living things that will need ongoing care and attention. It involves working with nature and with your hands in the soil. This can be very therapeutic. Terrariums create their own rain storm on the sides of the bottle so the little ecosystem can provide an ever-changing observation station. This task requires fine motor skills with a heavy cognitive component and problem-solving skills to determine how to plant properly so the plants will survive and flourish.

This project may enhance performance in the following component areas:

Motor Components

- Fine motor abilities of the hand
- Coordination of the hand/eye
- Use of hands bilaterally

Cognitive Components

- Organizational abilities
- Problem-solving abilities
- Ability to plan
- Concentration
- Attention to task
- Sequencing ability
- Decision-making skills

Perceptual Components

- Eye-hand coordination
- Awareness of spatial relation
- Tactile awareness in the hands
- Motor planning of hands and upper extremities

- Constructional praxia

Emotional Components

- Independence
- Self-esteem

Social Components

- Responsibility
- Ability to work alone

Adaptations

- Position required—sitting upright or standing
- Allows for repetition of hand and finger motions
- Can be done individually
- Design could incorporate some individual cultural values

GENERAL INFORMATION

1. Age—teenager to adult
2. Cost—expensive, but broken down by number of clinic treatments, it is reasonable
3. Visual requirements—good visual acuity or corrected with glasses
4. Instructions can be given verbally, written, or through demonstration

SUPPLIES

- Container with large opening is best for a beginner
- Potting soil
- Stones
- Charcoal
- Gloves (optional)
- Straw, long stick, or fine dowel
- Decorative moss
- Plants or cuttings

PRECAUTIONS

This activity is dirty and messy. The glass bottle can be broken by dropping the stones into it. Avoid this by tipping the bottle and rolling the stones down to the bottom. Rearrange them once the bottle is turned upright. Not appropriate for clients with open wounds on the hands or forearm.

ACTIVITY GRADATION

The size of the top of the container will increase or decrease the degree of difficulty in this task.

NOTE Terrariums were first designed by a British surgeon, Dr. Nathaniel Ward, in 1832. He was studying moths and found that the soil in the bottom of the container with the moth started to grow a fern and some grass. He was so fascinated he started studying the growth of plants in closed containers. Terrariums are living things that provide pleasure by watching them grow. They even create their own daily rain storms. They require only a minimum of care and can last for years.

There is much written about terrariums and if you wish to learn more, the library can help you find many articles about terrariums. Listed below are the very basics to get started.

Client Information for Terrariums

SUPPLIES

- Container with large opening is best for a beginner
- Potting soil
- Stones
- Charcoal
- Gloves (optional)
- Straw, long stick, or fine dowel
- Decorative moss
- Plants or cuttings

INSTRUCTIONS

1. The container should be clean and dry.
2. The first, or bottom layer, should be a thin layer of moss. Place it upside down with the mossy part against the glass surface.
3. The second, or drainage layer, contains crushed charcoal sprinkled over the moss. Next add a layer of small pebbles or stones with some added charcoal on top.

4. The third layer is the soil. Soil is easily handled when slightly moist.

   Note: For the most pleasing effect, all of the potting materials, layers one to three, should not exceed one third the height of the container.

5. Add plants to the potting mixture. The tallest plants should be added first.
6. Remove the plants from their pots immediately before transplanting.
7. Gently loosen the root ball to free the plant. It is much easier to transplant through the bottle opening.
8. Position the plant at the soil depth equal to that of the pot it was in.
9. Press the soil firmly around each plant.

   Note: Each plant needs space around it to spread out and grow larger.

10. Arrange the plants in an asymmetrical (off-center) pattern. Try to have one focal point within the planting design.
11. Add decorative items such as driftwood, rocks, or ceramic animals to add interest to the design.

SOME HANDY INFORMATION

- Never put a finished terrarium in direct sunlight. The plants will burn in the sun.
- Do not use a tinted container, as the light source for the plants will not be sufficient.
- Choose plants that are in keeping with the size of the container.
- Turn the terrarium occasionally to keep the growth of the plants even.
- Distilled water is best for terrariums.
- Don't over water. Mold is the greatest enemy of terrariums.
- Plants can be cut back if they become overgrown.

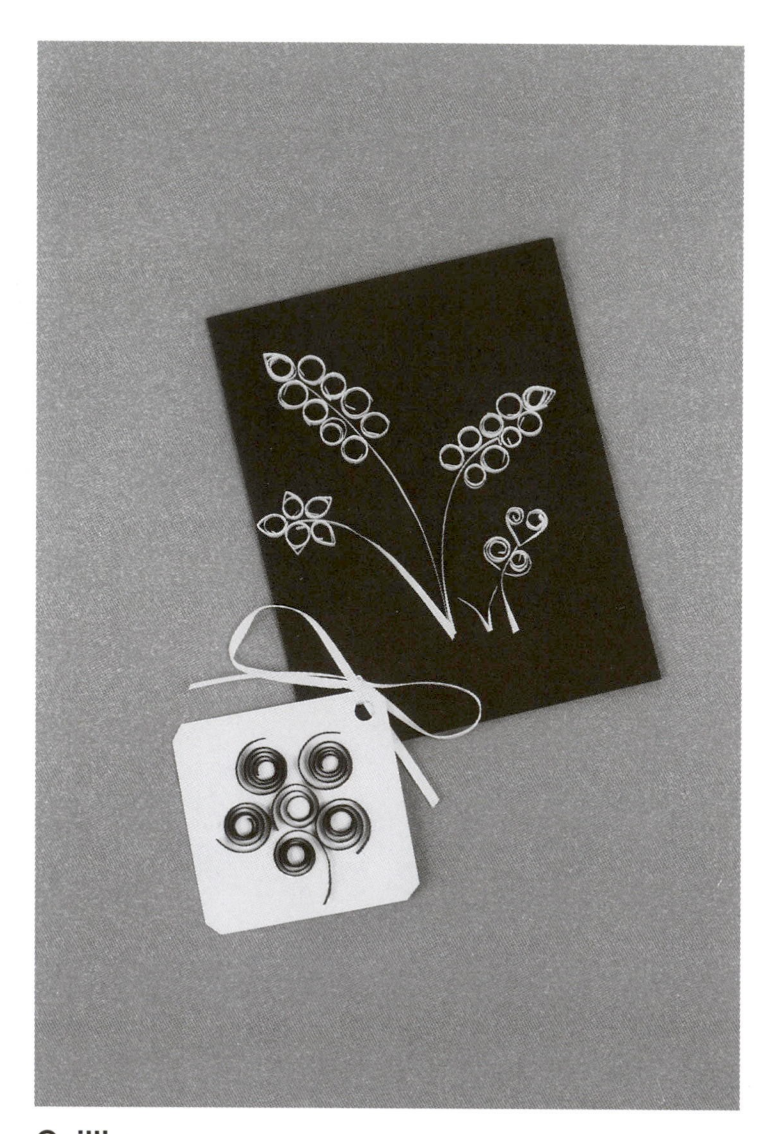

Quilling

Chapter 23

QUILLING

Therapist Information for Quilling

ACTIVITY ANALYSIS

Quilling is accomplished by rolling 1/8-inch-wide strips of paper into various shapes. These shapes can be used individually or in groups to form larger designs. Patterns can be designed and planned carefully or can be done as you work. This is an excellent fine motor task. It is also a good task for someone on bed rest.

This project may enhance performance in the following component areas:

Motor Components

- Fine motor abilities of the hand
- Coordination of the hand/arm
- Use of hands bilaterally

Cognitive Components

- Organizational abilities
- Ability to plan
- Concentration
- Attention to task
- Sequencing ability

Perceptual Components

- Awareness of spatial relations
- Tactile awareness in the hands

Emotional Components

- Independence
- Self-esteem

Social Components

- Ability to work alone

Adaptations

- Position required—sitting upright or reclining
- Allows for repetition of hand and finger motions
- High success rate
- Can vary from a structured to an unstructured activity
- Can be done individually
- Can be adapted for a group
- Design could incorporate some individual cultural values

GENERAL INFORMATION

1. Age—child through adult
2. Cost—minimal
3. Visual requirements—generally good visual acuity; however, tactile sense can assist with this project
4. Instructions can be given verbally, written, or through demonstration

SUPPLIES

- Glue
- Strips of paper 1/8-inch wide in various lengths, handmade or purchased
- Toothpicks or dowel rod with a slit in tip
- Scissors
- Tweezers (optional)

PRECAUTIONS

Precautions using sharp objects are necessary when using scissors. If the client has tendencies toward perfection, this may be a frustrating task to complete. It also may be difficult for clients with tremors.

ACTIVITY GRADATION

The number of colors of paper can vary as well as the size of design. The design can be planned or done spontaneously.

NOTE This project can be accomplished fairly quickly and can provide an attractive way to decorate cards or packages. Follow our design or plan one of your own. You can change the shape of the design by squeezing the coils in different ways.

Client Information for Quilling

SUPPLIES

- Glue
- Strips of paper 1/8-inch wide in various lengths, hand made or purchased
- Toothpicks or dowel rod with a slit in tip
- Scissors
- Tweezers (optional)

INSTRUCTIONS

1. Slit one end of a dowel or toothpick.
2. Place the end of one strip of paper into the slit.
3. Slowly turn the dowel or toothpick counter clockwise with one hand and pull slightly at the other end of the paper with your other hand to provide tension.
4. Roll the whole strip of paper evenly.
5. Squeeze the coil lightly before removing it from the dowel or toothpick. Note: The end of the paper can be left loose to uncoil or the end can be glued to the coil, depending on the effect desired.
6. Put a dot of glue at the end of the coil to secure it tightly.
7. Hold for several seconds to allow the glue to adhere properly.
8. Place the coils as shown in our sample.

   Note: Improvisation is encouraged. Coils can be squeezed to make tear drop or oval shapes if desired.

CORRECTING MISTAKES

The pieces can be moved before the glue dries. Once the glue has dried the card surface will be damaged if you try to remove it.

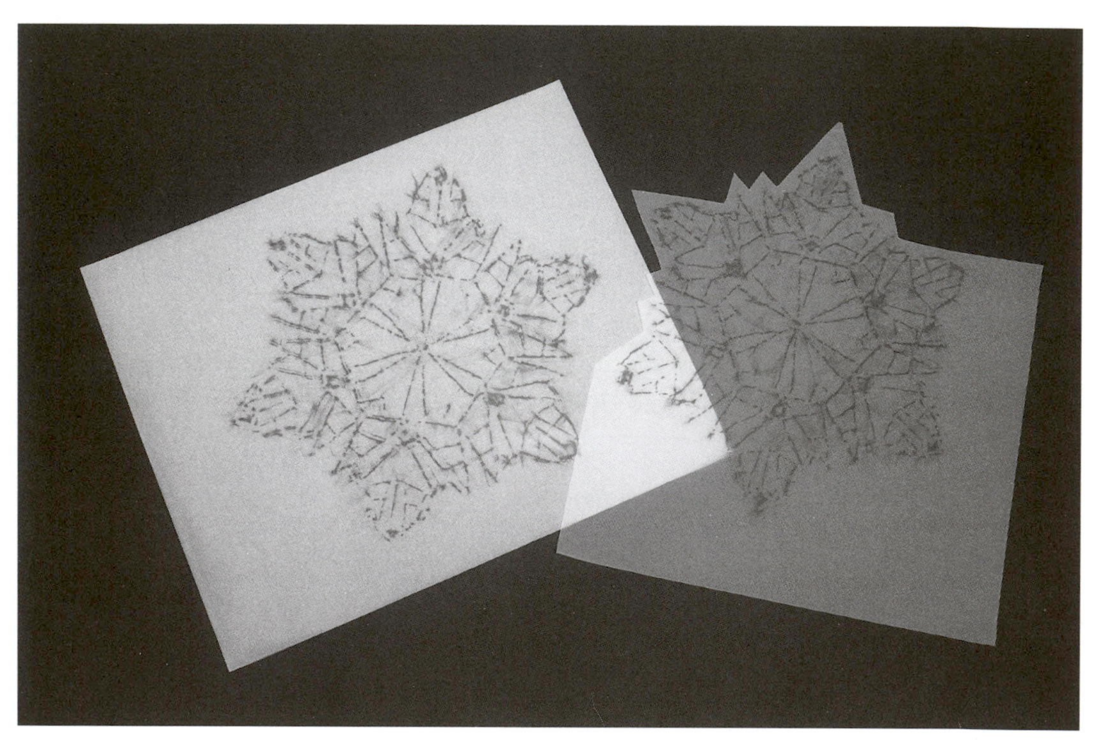

Rubbings

Chapter 24

RUBBINGS

Therapist Information for Rubbings

ACTIVITY ANALYSIS

Rubbings use both fine and gross motor skills and is a fun craft to use in conjunction with topographical orientation training. A scavenger-hunt-like game can be played by having the client do a rubbing of environmental patterns (i.e., grate covers or floor tiles from various locations) along a predetermined route to prove that he or she has found those locations.

Motor Components

- Fine motor abilities of the hand
- Coordination of the hand/arm
- Hand dominance
- Use of hands bilaterally
- Endurance
- Strength

Cognitive Components

- Organizational abilities
- Problem-solving abilities
- Ability to plan
- Concentration
- Attention to task
- Sequencing ability
- Decison-making skills

Perceptual Components

- Eye-hand coordination
- Tactile awareness in the hands
- Motor planning of hands and upper extremities

- Awareness of neglected side

Emotional Components

- Self-esteem

Social Components

- Ability to work alone

Adaptations

- Position required—sitting, kneeling, or standing. Some trunk-forward flexion is required.
- Allows for repetition of hand and finger motions
- Can be used for one-handed training, with use of adaptive equipment
- Can be done individually
- Design could incorporate some cultural values of an individual

GENERAL INFORMATION

1. Age—8 years through adult
2. Cost—inexpensive
3. Visual requirements—this craft can be performed by a client who is visually impaired
4. Instructions can be given verbally, written, or through demonstration

SUPPLIES

- Tracing paper
- Charcoal, chalk, or wax crayons
- Masking tape
- Spray fixative to keep rubbing from smearing

PRECAUTIONS

Do not let a topographically disoriented client follow the game route unescorted. A client who is tactically hypersensitive may need to wear gloves to dampen the tactile input through the fingers/hands.

ACTIVITY GRADATION

A beginner at this technique may wish to safely experiment with a manhole cover, a cornerstone of a building, or a plaque on the wall. Size of the rubbing can vary. Because most of the objects that would be worthy of doing a rubbing on are a distance from the clinic, travel to those locations is a consideration.

NOTE Rubbings are a time-honored craft. The earliest known rubbings date back to the second century A.D. in China when damp paper was placed against stone carvings and rubbed with ink to reproduce the images. It is a way to take a permanent remembrance of an immovable object (i.e., a historic plaque or a tombstone engraving). The task is easily done using thin tracing paper and charcoal, chalk, or crayons. If done carefully, the rubbing can be framed to be used as a wall decoration in the home.

Client Information for Rubbings

SUPPLIES

- Tracing paper
- Charcoal, chalk, or wax crayons
- Masking tape
- Spray fixative to keep rubbing from smearing

INSTRUCTIONS

1. Find a suitable texture to transfer.
2. Lay the tracing paper over the design, trying to center the design within the dimensions of the paper size.
3. Use masking tape to secure the tracing paper over the design.
4. Hold the charcoal, chalk, or crayon so the broad side runs across the design.
5. Start at the center of the design and work outward.
6. Rub the charcoal, chalk, or crayon across the design using a slight downward pressure to transfer the design.
7. Go over the design as many times as you need to get a good impression transfer onto the paper.

   Note: You may need to do a practice rubbing first to get the feel for this technique. Bring several sheets of paper with which to experiment.

8. Use spray fixative to keep the rubbing from smearing. Follow label directions.

CORRECTING MISTAKES

Mistakes cannot be corrected. Start over with a new sheet of paper.

CARE OF PROJECT

To keep project from smearing, spray with commercial fixative. The project can be dusted once it is framed. Do not apply water to finished project.

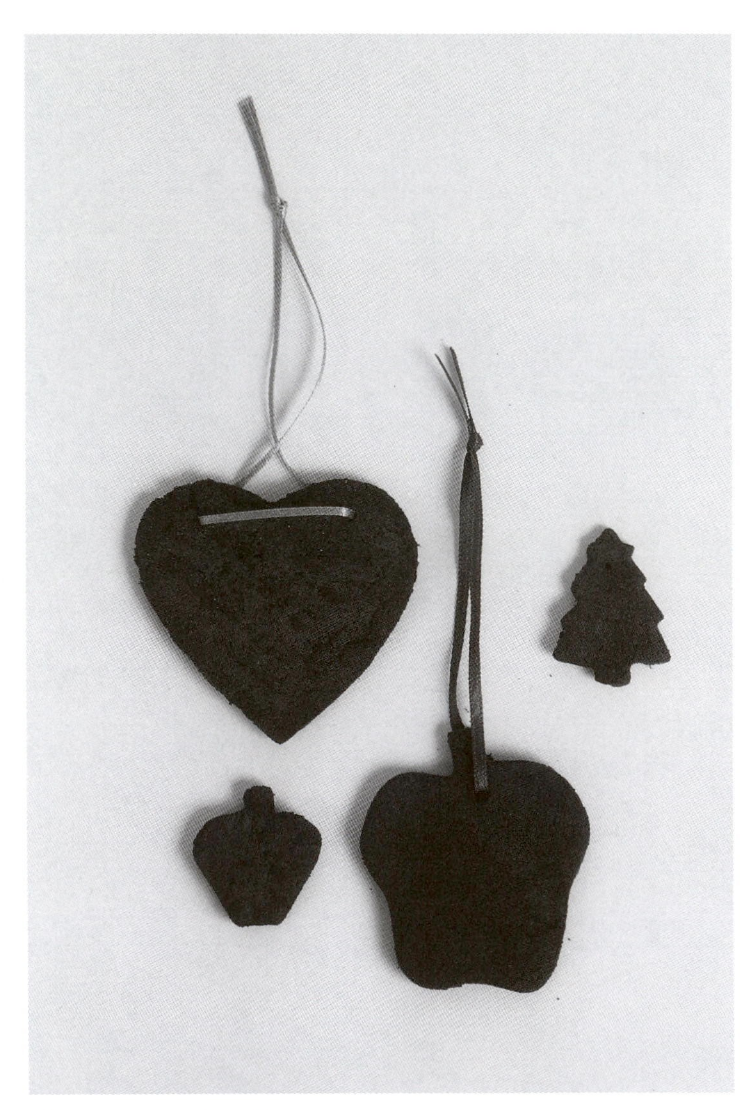

Cinnamon Cut Outs

Chapter 25

CINNAMON CUT OUTS

Therapist Information for Cinnamon Cut Outs

ACTIVITY ANALYSIS

This is a simple, fast, and good smelling craft. The cut-out shapes can be made into ornaments, used as decorations on wreaths or presents, or used as simple wall hangings. They can be completed in approximately ½-hour sessions, excluding drying time. This is an excellent group project. It can be done any time of year, but is especially useful in the fall or at holiday time. This craft is excellent for providing olfactory stimulation and increased tactile input. An excellent craft for clients with visual impairments.

This project may enhance performance in the following component areas:

Motor Components

- Fine motor abilities of the hand
- Coordination of the hand/arm
- Hand dominance
- Use of hands bilaterally
- Strength

Cognitive Components

- Attention to task
- Sequencing ability
- Decision-making skills

Perceptual Components

- Tactile awareness in the hands
- Motor planning of hands and upper extremities

Emotional Components

- Self-esteem
- Release of negative feelings

Social Components

- Comfort level in group settings
- Sociability in new situations

Adaptations

- Position required—sitting upright or standing
- Allows for repetition of hand and finger motions
- Can be used for one-handed training, with use of adaptive equipment
- High success rate
- Can be done individually
- Can be adapted for a group

GENERAL INFORMATION

1. Age—child through adult
2. Cost—inexpensive
3. Visual requirements—this craft can be performed by clients who are visually impaired
4. Instructions can be given verbally, written, or through demonstration

SUPPLIES

- 4.12 ounces of cinnamon
- ¾ cup applesauce
- Variety of cookie cutters
- Rolling pin
- Cookie cooling rack
- Vegetable spray
- Toothpicks
- Spatula

PRECAUTIONS

Clients with allergies or respiratory diseases may find the intense cinnamon smell irritating. Tactile-hypersensitive clients may need to wear gloves to dampen the input. Cookie cutters have sharp edges and should be used with supervision.

ACTIVITY GRADATION

The dough can be pre-mixed for a group to use, and it can be rolled out by the therapist, so only the client cuts it.

NOTE This craft can be done in a short amount of time. The smell of cinnamon is sweet as you work with the dough and it will continue to smell after the shapes are dry. Choose your favorite cookie cutter shapes or make up an original shape. The cinnamon cut outs make wonderful gifts or pretty additons to gift wrappings or they can be hung in a room to add a pleasant smell.

Client Information for Cinnamon Cut Outs

SUPPLIES

- 4.12 ounces of cinnamon
- ¾ cup applesauce
- Variety of cookie cutters
- Rolling pin
- Cookie cooling rack
- Vegetable spray
- Toothpicks
- Spatula

INSTRUCTIONS

1. In a bowl, mix cinnamon and applesauce well with a spoon or with hands.

   Note: There is an intense cinnamon smell until the cinnamon is all mixed into the applesauce.

2. Spray vegetable oil on the work surface to keep dough from sticking.
3. Remove half of the dough from the bowl and place on work surface.
4. Spray vegetable oil on the rolling pin.
5. Roll out the dough until it is ¼- to ½-inch thick.

   Note: If too thin, the shapes may curl during drying.

6. Choose a cookie cutter shape.

7. Press cookie cutter into rolled dough.
8. Remove cut out shape with a spatula and carefully place on the cookie rack for drying.
9. Air dry for approximately 48 hours.
10. Turn shapes over occasionally while drying.

CORRECTING MISTAKES

If shapes break apart while removing from the work surface, knead dough back into a ball and roll out again and re-cut.

CARE OF PROJECT

Do not immerse in water—ornaments are fairly fragile. Handle with care.

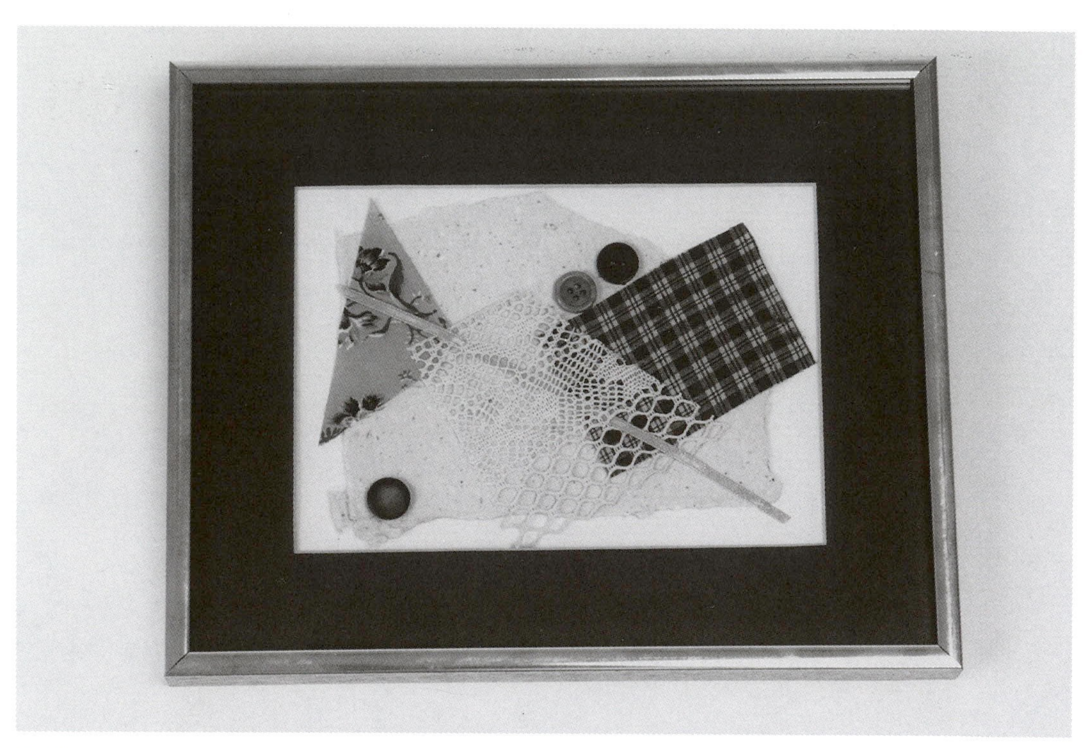

Collage

Chapter 26

COLLAGE

Therapist Information for Collage

ACTIVITY ANALYSIS

Collage is an interesting activity that can use a variety of media to create a pleasing wall decoration—cloth, paper, ink, pictures, shells. The possibilities are endless. This is an excellent task for problem solving and increasing organizational skills. This craft allows for freedom in final design and in choices of objects to be used to complete the design.

This project may enhance performance in the following component areas:

Motor Components

- Fine motor abilities of the hand
- Coordination of the hand/arm
- Hand dominance
- Use of hands bilaterally

Cognitive Components

- Organizational abilities
- Problem-solving abilities
- Ability to plan
- Concentration
- Attention to task
- Decision-making skills

Perceptual Components

- Eye-hand coordination
- Awareness of spatial relations
- Tactile awareness in the hands
- Constructional praxia

Emotional Components

- Self-esteem
- Independence

Social Components

- Ability to work alone

Adaptations

- Position required—sitting upright, reclining, or standing
- Can be used for one-handed training with use of adaptive equipment
- High success rate
- Can vary from a structured to an unstructured activity
- Can be done individually
- Can be adapted for a group
- Design could incorporate some cultural values of an individual

GENERAL INFORMATION

1. Age—child through adult
2. Cost—frame and matting vary in price, but can be commercially purchased, design itself is inexpensive
3. Visual requirements—good visual acuity or corrected with glasses
4. Instructions can be given verbally or through demonstration. Specific written instructions are very difficult because of the variety of media possibilities.

SUPPLIES

- Base cardboard
- Scissors
- Glue
- Frame
- Mat
- Ribbons
- Papers
- Fabrics
- Pictures
- Flat odds and ends

PRECAUTIONS

Precautions with sharp objects are necessary when using scissors. If a client is in manic phase of bipolar disorder, the size of the project needs to be monitored by therapist. Not for clients who eat non-food items (PICA).

ACTIVITY GRADATION

The amount of media choices can be varied to expand or limit decision making. The size of the frame can be varied to increase complexity of the task.

This task can be used in conjunction with paper-making task which is included in this text to provide ongoing group experiences and increased complexity.

NOTE This project can use personal items that hold significance, such as favorite photographs, fabrics from old, cherished cloths (i.e., prom or wedding dress) or handmade paper. The types of media that could be used are endless. The task allows you to arrange the items in a pleasing grouping, framed to last.

Client Information for Collage

SUPPLIES

- Base cardboard
- Scissors
- Glue
- Frame
- Mat
- Ribbons
- Papers
- Fabrics
- Pictures
- Flat odds and ends

INSTRUCTIONS

1. Choose a decorative piece of cardboard for backing and cut to size of frame.
2. Choose variety of meaningful flat objects, pictures, or fabrics.
3. Experiment with arranging objects in a pleasing design that will fit into

the open space in the mat (which is a smaller dimension than the frame).

4. Once desired arrangement is achieved, carefully spot glue pieces to background cardboard.
5. Lay mat over design.
6. Lay glass from frame on top of the mat. Be careful not to cut fingers on edges of glass.
7. Place frame on top of glass.
8. Follow specific directions that came with the frame to hold the picture securely.

CORRECTING MISTAKES

Experiment with design as long as needed to be pleased with it. Once glued in place it cannot be changed.

CARE OF PROJECT

Dust only. Do not immerse in water.

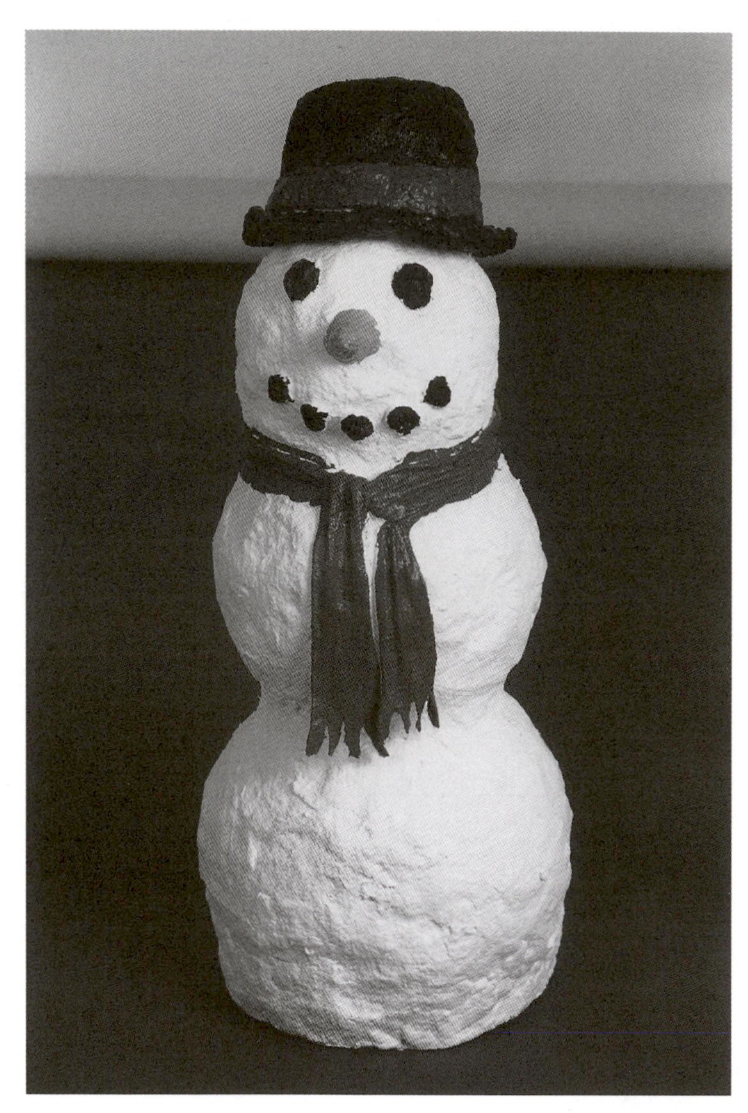

Papier-Mâché

Chapter 27

PAPIER-MÂCHÉ

Therapist Information for Papier-Mâché

ACTIVITY ANALYSIS

The "Instant Papier-Mâché" from the S&S Arts and Crafts catalog is an excellent project for a client who needs to strengthen the intrinsic muscles of the hand or needs to work on increasing sensory input and feedback from the hand. Warm water can be used to mix the Instant Papier-Mâché to provide a soothing environment for arthritic hands. This material can be cooled in the refrigerator, however, if a cold medium is desired.

Traditional armature (internal structure) used for papier-mâché could be clothes hangers, chicken wire, or cardboard boxes. Any internal structure must be able to bear the wet weight of the papier-mâché materials.

The sample project was picked because it is a high success project that can be completed quickly. Armature is three Styrofoam™ balls with the edges cut off so they will not roll. The Styrofoam balls are glued together.

This project may enhance performance in the following component areas:

Motor Components

- Fine motor abilities of the hand
- Coordination of the hand/arm
- Hand dominance
- Use of hands bilaterally
- Endurance
- Strength

Cognitive Components

- Ability to plan
- Attention to task
- Sequencing ability
- Decision-making skills

Perceptual Components
- Eye-hand coordination
- Awareness of spatial relations
- Tactile awareness in the hands
- Motor planning of hands and upper extremities
- Constructional praxia

Emotional Components
- Independence
- Self-esteem

Social Components
- Comfort level in group settings
- Sociability in new situations
- Ability to work alone

Adaptations
- Position required—sitting upright or standing
- Allows for repetition of hand and finger motions
- Can be used for one-handed training with use of adaptive equipment
- High success rate
- Can vary from a structured to an unstructured activity
- Can be done individually
- Can be adapted for a group
- Design could incorporate some individual cultural values

GENERAL INFORMATION

1. Age—teenager through adult
2. Cost—moderate
3. Visual requirements—fair visual acuity or corrected with glasses
4. Instructions can be given verbally, written, or through demonstration

SUPPLIES

- Large mixing bowl
- Package of Celluclay
- S&S Arts and Crafts catalog No. PL-60A, Instant Papier-Mâché (1-pound package) (1-800-243-9232)
- Four cups warm water

- Three Styrofoam balls (6 inches, 8 inches, and 10 inches)
- Glue
- Toothpick
- Gesso
- Acrylic paints
- Paint brush
- 32-ounce size plastic glass
- Electric knife (optional)
- Waxed paper to use a work surface
- Cookie cooling rack to set pieces on to dry

PRECAUTIONS

This task is very dusty at first. The mixing with water is not for someone with respiratory disease, unless wearing an isolation mask. This project has an odor until dry. Contraindicated for any client who would eat non-food items (PICA).

ACTIVITY GRADATION

The instant papier-mâché can be pre-mixed for use with respiratory clients. The task can be made easier by using smaller Styrofoam balls. (The detail work on the snowman can be omitted.)

NOTE Papier-mâché is an interesting creative process. In the task shown in this text, you take a package containing paper dust, add water, and use the mixture to create a seasonal decoration. This mixture can be used to create other sculptures or containers (i.e., flower pots or boxes) of your choice. No special tools are needed. The finished project can be painted. The project will be a keepsake for years to come.

Client Information for Papier-Mâché

SUPPLIES

- Large mixing bowl
- Package of Celluclay
- S&S Arts and Crafts catalog No. PL-60A, Instant Papier-Mâché (1-pound package) (1-800-243-9232)
- Four cups warm water
- Three Styrofoam balls (6 inches, 8 inches, and 10 inches)

- Glue
- Toothpick
- Gesso
- Acrylic paints
- Paint brush
- 32-ounce size plastic glass
- Electric knife (optional)
- Waxed paper to use a work surface
- Cookie cooling rack to set pieces on to dry

INSTRUCTIONS

1. Use an electric carving knife to cut off the bottom and top of the 10-inch Styrofoam ball.
2. Use an electric carving knife to cut off the bottom and top of the 8-inch Styrofoam ball.
3. Use an electric knife to cut off the bottom of the 6-inch Styrofoam ball.
4. Break three toothpicks in half. Insert three halves into the top of the 10-inch ball.
5. Put glue all around the flattened area and a little on each toothpick.
6. Place the 8-inch ball (one of the flattened areas) over the toothpicks and glue and press the two balls together. You now have the bottom two thirds of the snowman.
7. Place the remaining three halves of the toothpicks into the flattened area on top of the 8-inch ball.
8. Put the glue all over the flattened area and a little on each toothpick.
9. Place the flattened area of the 6-inch ball over the toothpicks and glue onto the top of the 8-inch ball and press together. You now have the whole snowman support.
10. Let glue dry for 1 to 2 hours.

    Note: Step 11 is very dusty. You may need to cover your mouth with an iso-mask or turn your head sideways.

11. Mix the Instant Papier-Mâché in a large bowl, adding 4 cups of very warm water.
12. Mix or knead with your hands until well mixed.
13. Take small clumps of the mixture and pat it smoothly and evenly onto the Styrofoam frame.
14. The thickness of the Instant Papier-mâché should be about 1/8-inch thick all over the Styrofoam.
15. Continue steps 13 and 14 until the entire Styrofoam snowman is covered.
16. Make small balls for the eyes and smile to look like coal. They do not need to be very big. Push the pieces into place.
17. Form a small "carrot" and put in place for the nose.
18. A scarf for the snowman can be formed as desired or a piece of cloth can be substituted later to finish the design.
19. Form the hat over the bottom of the 32-ounce cup. Cover about 4 inches of the bottom of the cup.
20. To form the brim of the hat, pat some of the mixture onto a piece of waxed paper, forming a 5-inch diameter circle shape.
21. Put all pieces of the project in a safe place to dry for 2–3 days.
22. Paint the entire surface of the snowman with gesso. This is a primer coat that will make the acrylic paint cover and look better.
23. Paint with acrylic paint colors of your choice.

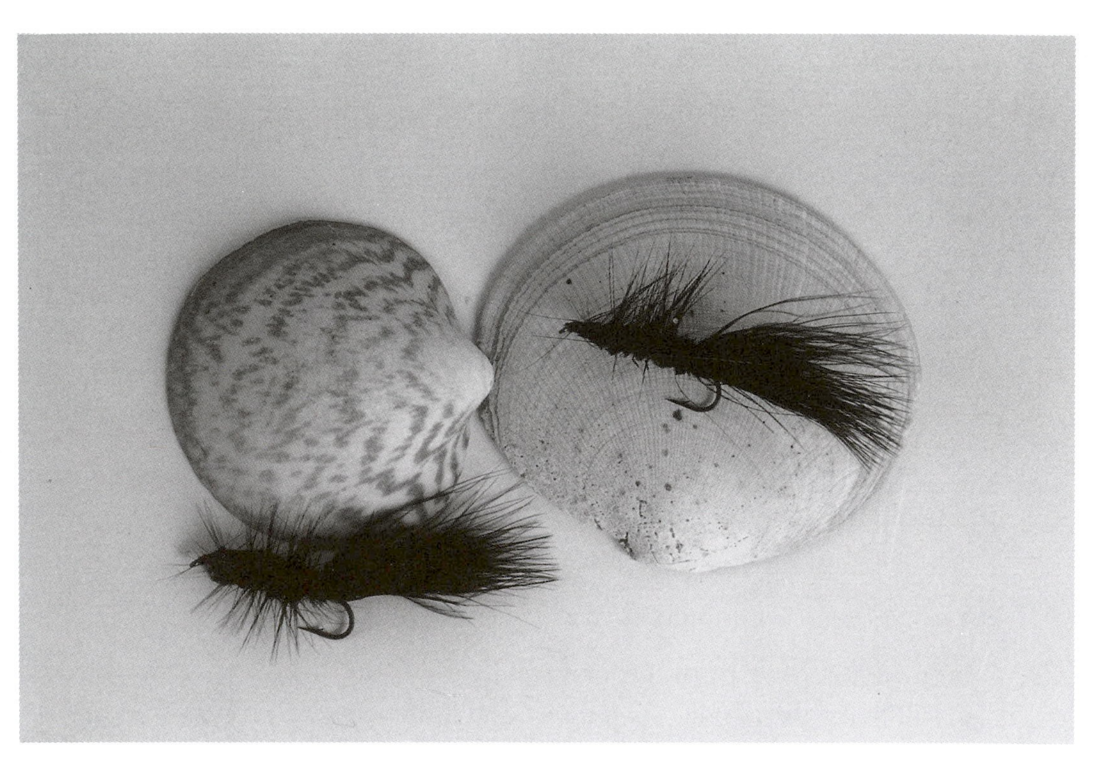

Fly Tying

Chapter 28

FLY TYING

Therapist Information for Fly Tying

ACTIVITY ANALYSIS

Fly Tying is a craft and an art. It has many spiritual aspects for the fisherman who creates his or her own flies. There are recipes for making flies just as there are recipes for making cakes. The easiest flies to do as a beginner are "wet flies." A Wooly Bugger fly is shown as our sample. All the steps in tying any fly are present, and the information can be generalized without too much difficulty.

Fly Tying is an expensive craft activity to start, but relatively inexpensive once you have the vice and basic tools and materials. Fly Tying is an excellent activity for someone who doesn't do crafts, but does fish. The task includes problem solving, spatial relations, fine motor, and coordination.

This project may enhance performance in the following component areas:

Motor Components

- Fine motor abilities of the hand
- Coordination of the hand/arm
- Use of hands bilaterally
- Endurance

Cognitive Components

- Organizational abilities
- Problem-solving abilities
- Ability to plan
- Coordination
- Attention to task
- Sequencing ability
- Decision-making skills

Perceptual Components

- Eye-hand coordination
- Awareness of spatial relations
- Tactile awareness of the hands
- Motor planning of the hands and upper extremities
- Constructional praxia

Emotional Components

- Independence
- Self-esteem

Social Components

- Ability to work alone

Adaptations

- Position required—sitting upright
- Allows for repetition of hand and finger motions
- Can be done individually

GENERAL INFORMATION

1. Age—adult
2. Cost—expensive if initially buying supplies, fairly inexpensive if supplies available
3. Visual requirements—good visual acuity or corrected with glasses
4. Instructions may be given verbally, written, or through demonstration. This craft is much easier if it is shown by demonstration before the individual tries it on his or her own.

SUPPLIES

The sample presented is a Wooly Bugger Fly.

- Number 4 hook
- Special tying thread (black)
- Grizzly Hackle Feathers
- Deer hair
- Vice and stand (vices can be purchased to use a four-finger grasp, a lateral pinch, or a three-jaw-chuck pinchbased on needs of the client)
- Thread bobbin
- Hackle pliers
- Small bit of eraser

- Lead wire (16 gauge)
- Small scissors
- Hair stacker (optional)
- Chenille (black)
- Head cement

PRECAUTIONS

The hooks are sharp. A small eraser can be put over the tip to protect fingers and thread. Small scissors are used so precautions should be observed. This activity may be difficult for clients with tremors or severe incoordination and painful small hand joints.

ACTIVITY GRADATION

There are an infinite variety of "flies," both wet and dry, and there are a multitude of books available on fly tying.

NOTE For some fishermen, tying flies is a spiritual experience and requires adherence to the "ritual" of tying flies. (A good basic kit is helpful because it provides a variety of materials.)

Client Information for Fly Tying

SUPPLIES

The sample presented is a Wooly Bugger Fly.

- Number 4 hook
- Special tying thread (black)
- Grizzly Hackle Feathers
- Deer hair
- Vice and stand (vices can be purchased to use a four-finger grasp, a lateral pinch, or a three-jaw-chuck pinch based on needs of the client)
- Thread bobbin
- Hackle pliers
- Small bit of eraser
- Lead wire (16 gauge)
- Small scissors
- Hair stacker (optional)

- Chenille (black)
- Head cement

INSTRUCTIONS

1. Place the lower part of the hook into the vice (Figure 28-1).
2. Place a small eraser on the end of the hook to protect fingers and thread.
3. Wrap the hook shaft with thread (wrap away from you) from middle of shank to eye of hook.
4. Tie off with "half hitch" knot and clip with small scissors.
5. Wrap a 16-gauge wire around center third of the shaft and push both ends of the wire toward the center to compress it (Figure 28-2).
6. Cut off extra wire with small scissors.
7. Wrap thread over lead wire to tie it down to shaft of hook and keep it in place.
8. Cut some deer hairs—about 3 times the distance between the hook and the shaft (Figure 28-3).
9. Pinch gently and tie deer hairs above the hook by wrapping half the hairs with thread to secure it (Figure 28-4).

   Note: The other half of the deer hairs will hang off the back to form the "fly tail."
10. Cut a piece of chenille—long enough to wrap 15 times around the hook.
11. Pull off the end chenille pieces to expose about ½ inch of the thread.
12. Tie down the chenille end with thread.
13. Wrap chenille around the hook 15 times—moving from tail end to eye end of the hook.
14. Tie down securely with thread.
15. Take a 3-inch grizzly hackle feather and pluck off some feathers at the end to expose about ½ inch of the stem of the feather.
16. Tie the stem end down securely at the tail end of the fly (Figure 28-5).

Figure 28-6

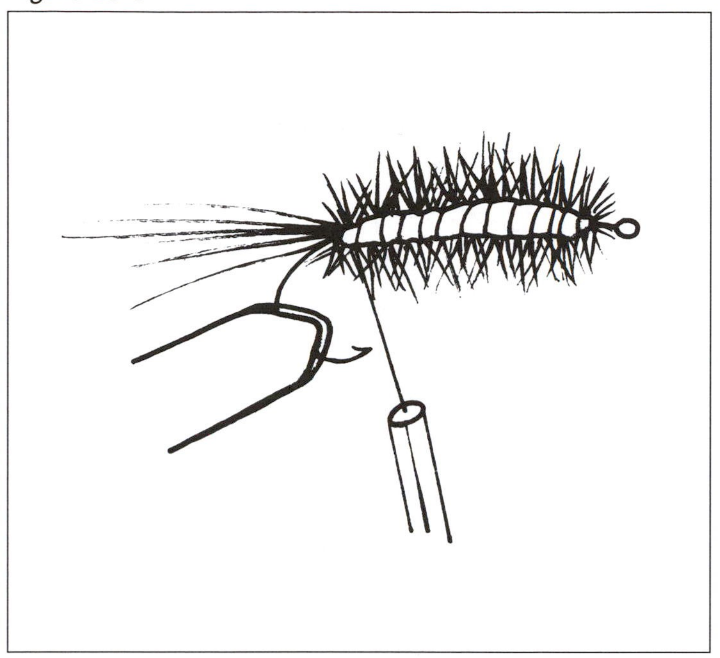

Figure 28-7

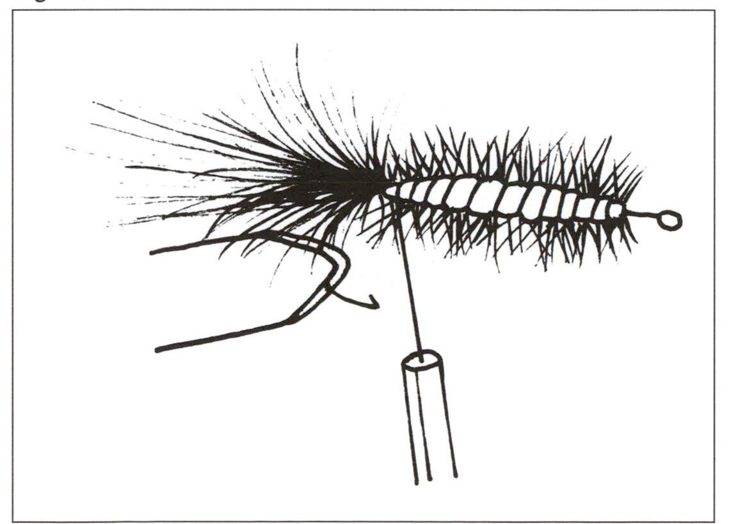

Figure 28-4

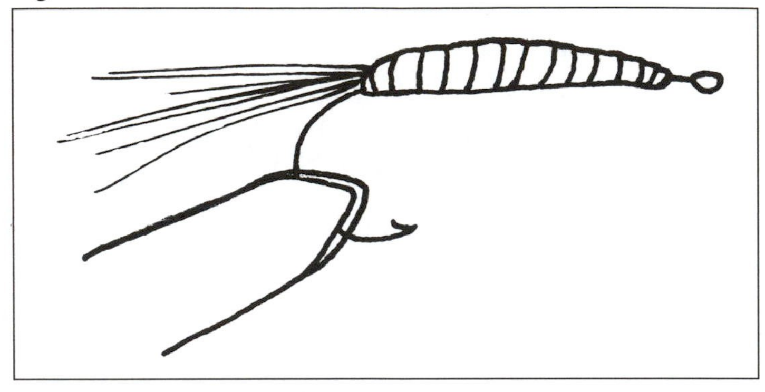

Figure 28-5

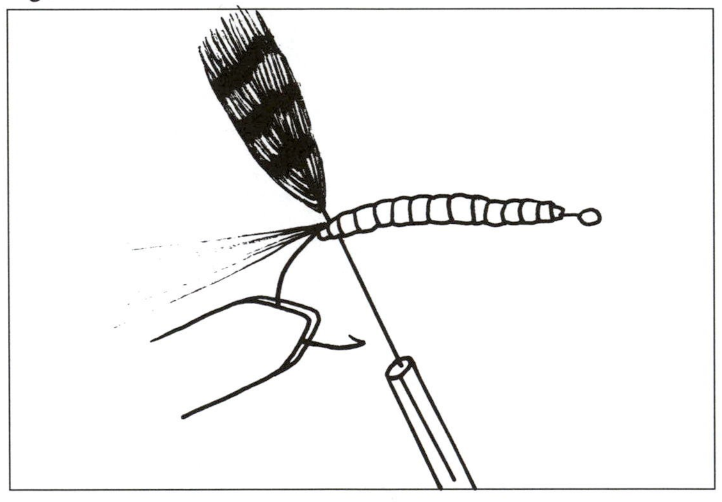

Figure 28-2

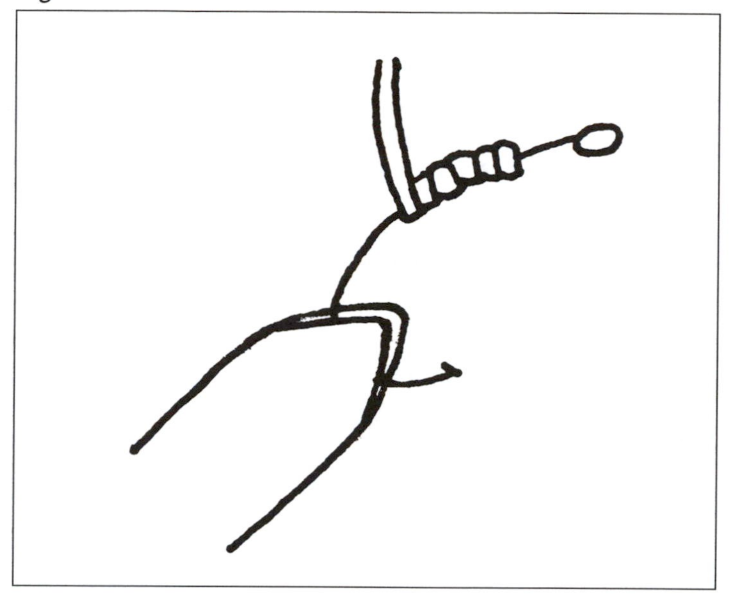

Figure 28-3

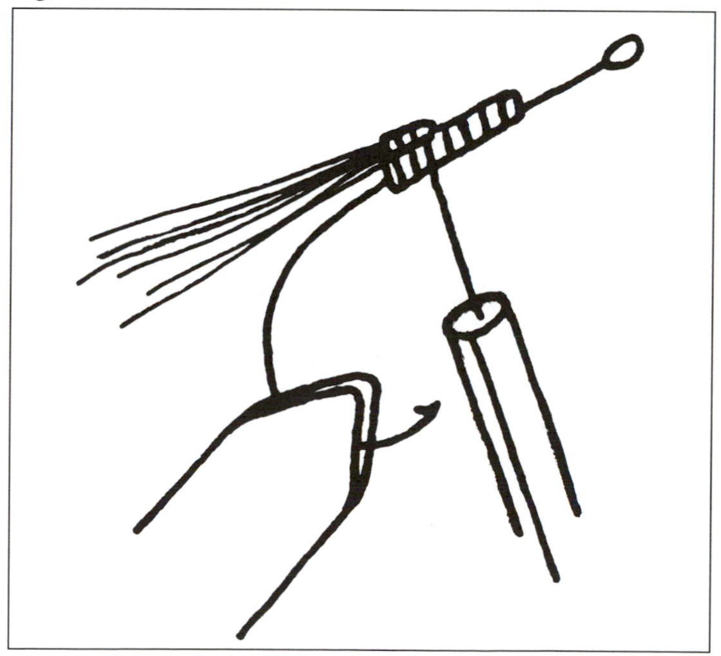

17. Pinch the end of the feather in the hackle plyers and wrap it so that the stem of the feather goes between the chenille "bumps" (Figure 28-6).

    Note: As you wrap the hackle feather, it will separate and look very "feathery" along the "body" of the fly. This is called Palmering (Figure 28-7).

18. Tie down the eye end of the hackle feather.
19. Tie off head of the fly with about three "half-hitch" knots.
20. Put a drop of head cement on the end of the string to secure.

Your fly should now be complete and ready to catch fish.

CORRECTING MISTAKES

If you make a mistake, you just start over and try again.

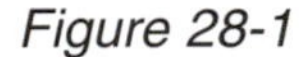

Figure 28-1

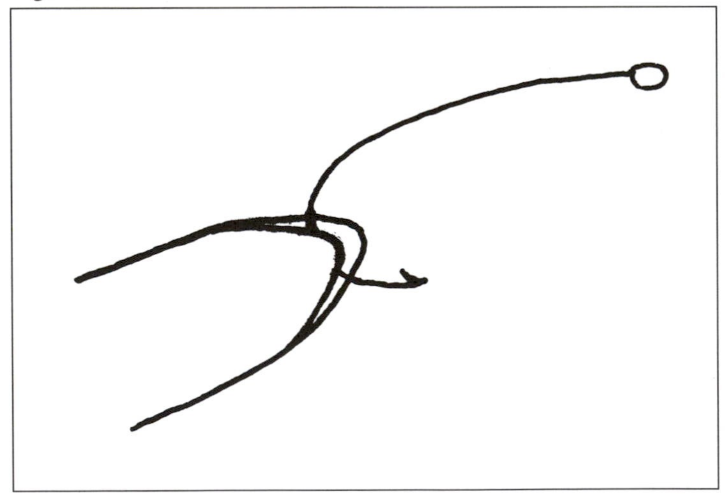

Eye-hand coordination: Integrated use of visual and motor response to achieve a result/action.

Fine motor abilities: Skill of using the hand/fingers for precise prehension, primarily using the thumb, index, and middle fingers.

Independence: Skill of working alone without intervention.

Motor planning of the hands and upper extremities: Ability to execute purposeful motor movements upon request.

Nondominant hand: Generally thought to be the upper extremity not used for precision during functional tasks, but as a stabilizing or assistive hand/arm (i.e., holds paper while writing with dominant hand)..

Organizational abilities: Skill of mental manipulation of information to see the parts of a given task and sequence them appropriately.

Problem-solving abilities: Process of recognizing difficulties and evaluating options or strategies to accomplish a task.

Release of negative feelings: Use of motor activity to relieve emotional tension.

Responsibility: The act of being dependable or following through.

Self-esteem: Setting a high value or respect on one's own personal concept.

Sequencing abilities: Ability to prioritize steps of a task in the appropriate order.

Sociability with new situations: Increased comfort and appropriate social interaction in which novel tasks are introduced.

Strength: Maximum tension in a muscle or muscle group. Maximum maintained muscle contraction.

Tactile awareness in the hands: Ability of the hands to relate to the brain sensory information.

Use of the hands bilaterally: Ability to use both upper extremities together in a coordinated fashion.

Glossary of Terms

For the purposes of this text, we have defined the following terms, listed alphabetically by first word in the term.

Ability to plan: Skill of developing a method for accomplishing a specific task.

Ability to work alone: Skill of working with one's own resources, not relying on others.

Attention to task: Ability to maintain focus and follow the process of the task, regardless of external stimuli.

Awareness of neglected side: Ability to correctly perceive and interpret information from the affected side of the body or the environment surrounding it.

Awareness of spatial relations: Perception of objects in relation to each other or the client.

Changing hand dominance: Learned skill of using the nondominant upper extremity to accomplish a functional task (i.e., handwriting, feeding oneself).

Comfort level in a group setting: Lessening the anxiety in a situation with a number of individuals.

Concentration: Skill of directing attention to a specific object.

Constructional apraxia: Ability to build objects in three dimensional designs.

Coordination of the hand/arm: Ability to use multiple muscle groups throughout the upper extremity to smoothly perform tasks.

Decision-making skills: Ability to analyze and select between available options.

Endurance: Sustained energy output sufficient to complete a given activity.

Appendix A

Motor Components

Fine motor abilities of the hand

- Bargello
- Birdhouse Kit
- Cinnamon Cut Outs
- Collage
- Counted Cross-Stitch Towel
- Decoupage/Sponge Paint Flower Pot
- Dough Art
- Fly Tying
- Jewelry
- Latch Hook
- Leather Moccasins Kit
- Nail Art
- Needlepunch
- Original Copper Tooling
- Paper Making
- Paper Twist Basket
- Papier-Mâché
- Pressed Flower Cards
- Quilling
- Rubbings
- Snail Cribbage Board
- Sponge-Stamped T-shirt
- String Art
- Terrariums
- Wood Burning
- Wooden Train Kit
- Wreath Making
- Yarn Picture

Gross coordination of the hand/arm

Bargello
Birdhouse Kit
Cinnamon Cut Outs
Collage
Counted Cross-Stitch Towel
Decoupage/Sponge Paint Flower Pot
Dough Art
Fly Tying
Latch Hook
Leather Moccasins Kit
Nail Art
Needlepunch
Original Copper Tooling
Paper Twist Basket
Papier-Mâché
Quilling
Rubbings
Snail Cribbage Board
Sponge-Stamped T-shirt
String Art
Terrariums
Wood Burning
Wooden Train Kit
Wreath Making
Yarn Picture

Hand dominance

Bargello
Birdhouse Kit
Cinnamon Cut Outs
Collage
Counted Cross-Stitch Towel
Decoupage/Sponge Paint Flower Pot
Dough Art
Nail Art
Needlepunch

Original Copper Tooling
Paper Making
Paper Twist Basket
Papier-Mâché
Pressed Flower Cards
Rubbings
Sponge-Stamped T-shirt
Wood Burning
Wreath Making
Yarn Picture

Use of hands bilaterally

Bargello
Birdhouse Kit
Cinnamon Cut Outs
Collage
Decoupage/Sponge Paint Flower Pot
Dough Art
Fly Tying
Jewelry
Latch Hook
Leather Moccasins Kit
Nail Art
Needlepunch
Paper Making
Papier-Mâché
Quilling
Rubbings
Snail Cribbage Board
String Art
Terrariums
Wooden Train Kit
Wreath Making
Yarn Picture

Endurance building

- Bargello
- Birdhouse Kit
- Counted Cross-Stitch Towel
- Decoupage/Sponge Paint Flower Pot
- Dough Art
- Fly Tying
- Latch Hook
- Leather Moccasins Kit
- Nail Art
- Needlepunch
- Paper Twist Basket
- Papier-Mâché
- Rubbings
- Snail Cribbage Board
- Sponge-Stamped T-shirt
- Wooden Train Kit
- Wreath Making

Strengthening

- Birdhouse Kit
- Cinnamon Cut Outs
- Dough Art
- Jewelry
- Latch Hook
- Leather Moccasins Kit
- Nail Art
- Original Copper Tooling
- Paper Making
- Paper Twist Basket
- Papier-Mâché
- Pressed Flower Cards
- Rubbings
- Snail Cribbage Board
- String Art
- Wood Burning
- Wreath Making

Appendix B

Cognitive Components

Organizational abilities

Collage
Counted Cross-Stitch Towel
Decoupage/Sponge Paint Flower Pot
Fly Tying
Jewelry
Latch Hook
Nail Art
Needlepunch
Original Copper Tooling
Paper Twist Basket
Pressed Flower Cards
Quilling
Rubbings
Snail Cribbage Board
Sponge-Stamped T-shirt
String Art
Terrariums
Wood Burning
Wooden Train Kit
Wreath Making
Yarn Picture

Problem-solving abilities

Birdhouse Kit
Collage
Decoupage/Sponge Paint Flower Pot
Fly Tying

Jewelry
Latch Hook
Leather Moccasins Kit
Nail Art
Needlepunch
Original Copper Tooling
Paper Twist Basket
Pressed Flower Cards
Rubbings
Snail Cribbage Board
Sponge-Stamped T-shirt
String Art
Terrariums
Wood Burning
Wooden Train Kit
Wreath Making
Yarn Picture

Planning ability

Bargello
Birdhouse Kit
Collage
Decoupage/Sponge Paint Flower Pot
Fly Tying
Jewelry
Latch Hook
Nail Art
Needlepunch
Original Copper Tooling
Paper Twist Basket
Papier-Mâché
Pressed Flower Cards
Quilling
Rubbings
Snail Cribbage Board
Sponge-Stamped T-shirt
String Art
Terrariums

Wood Burning
Wooden Train Kit
Wreath Making
Yarn Picture

Concentration skills

Bargello
Collage
Counted Cross-Stitch Towel
Decoupage/Sponge Paint Flower Pot
Dough Art
Fly Tying
Jewelry
Latch Hook
Leather Moccasins Kit
Nail Art
Needlepunch
Original Copper Tooling
Paper Twist Basket
Pressed Flower Cards
Quilling
Rubbings
Sponge-Stamped T-shirt
String Art
Terrariums
Wood Burning
Wooden Train Kit
Wreath Making

Attention to task

Bargello
Birdhouse Kit
Cinnamon Cut Outs
Collage
Counted Cross-Stitch Towel
Decoupage/Sponge Paint Flower Pot
Dough Art

Fly Tying
Jewelry
Nail Art
Needlepunch
Original Copper Tooling
Paper Twist Basket
Papier-Mâché
Quilling
Rubbings
Snail Cribbage Board
Sponge-Stamped T-shirt
String Art
Terrariums
Wood Burning
Wooden Train Kit
Wreath Making
Yarn Picture

Sequencing ability

Birdhouse Kit
Cinnamon Cut Outs
Counted Cross-Stitch Towel
Decoupage/Sponge Paint Flower Pot
Dough Art
Fly Tying
Jewelry
Leather Moccasins Kit
Needlepunch
Original Copper Tooling
Paper Making
Paper Twist Basket
Papier-Mâché
Pressed Flower Cards
Quilling
Rubbings
Snail Cribbage Board
Sponge-Stamped T-shirt
String Art

Terrariums
Wooden Train Kit
Wreath Making

Decision-making skills

Birdhouse Kit
Cinnamon Cut Outs
Collage
Counted Cross-Stitch Towel
Decoupage/Sponge Paint Flower Pot
Dough Art
Fly Tying
Jewelry
Needlepunch
Paper Twist Basket
Papier-Mâché
Rubbings
Snail Cribbage Board
Sponge-Stamped T-shirt
String Art
Terrariums
Wooden Train Kit
Wreath Making

Appendix C

Perceptual Components

Eye-hand coordination

Bargello
Birdhouse Kit
Collage
Counted Cross-Stitch Towel
Decoupage/Sponge Paint Flower Pot
Dough Art
Fly Tying
Jewelry
Latch Hook
Leather Moccasins Kit
Nail Art
Needlepunch
Original Copper Tooling
Paper Twist Basket
Papier-Mâché
Pressed Flower Cards
Quilling
Rubbings
Snail Cribbage Board
Sponge-Stamped T-shirt
String Art
Terrariums
Wood Burning
Wooden Train Kit
Wreath Making
Yarn Picture

Awareness of spatial relations

Bargello
Birdhouse Kit
Collage
Counted Cross-Stitch Towel
Decoupage/Sponge Paint Flower Pot
Fly Tying
Jewelry
Latch Hook
Nail Art
Needlepunch
Original Copper Tooling
Paper Twist Basket
Papier-Mâché
Pressed Flower Cards
Quilling
Snail Cribbage Board
Sponge-Stamped T-shirt
String Art
Terrariums
Wood Burning
Wooden Train Kit
Wreath Making
Yarn Picture

Tactile awareness in the hands

Bargello
Birdhouse Kit
Cinnamon Cut Outs
Collage
Dough Art
Fly Tying
Jewelry
Latch Hook
Leather Moccasins Kit
Nail Art
Needlepunch

Original Copper Tooling
Paper MakingPaper Twist Basket
Papier-Mâché
Quilling
Rubbings
Snail Cribbage Board
Sponge-Stamped T-shirt
String Art
Terrariums
Wooden Train Kit
Wreath Making
Yarn Picture

Motor planning of the hands and upper extremities

Bargello
Birdhouse Kit
Cinnamon Cut Outs
Counted Cross-Stitch Towel
Decoupage/Sponge Paint Flower Pot
Dough Art
Fly Tying
Jewelry
Latch Hook
Leather Moccasins Kit
Nail Art
Needlepunch
Original Copper Tooling
Paper Making
Paper Twist Basket
Papier-Mâché
Pressed Flower Cards
Rubbings
Snail Cribbage Board
Sponge-Stamped T-shirt
String Art
Terrariums
Wood Burning
Wooden Train Kit

Wreath Making
Yarn Picture

Awareness of neglected side

Latch Hook
Paper Making
Rubbings

Constructional praxia

Bargello
Birdhouse Kit
Collage
Fly Tying
Jewelry
Leather Moccasins Kit
Paper Twist Baskets
Papier-Mâché
Snail Cribbage Board
Terrariums
Wooden Train Kit

Appendix D

Emotional Components

Independence

Bargello
Birdhouse Kit
Collage
Counted Cross-Stitch Towel
Decoupage/Sponge Paint Flower Pot
Dough Art
Fly Tying
Jewelry
Latch Hook
Leather Moccasins Kit
Nail Art
Needlepunch
Original Copper Tooling
Paper Twist Basket
Papier-Mâché
Pressed Flower Cards
Quilling
Snail Cribbage Board
String Art
Terrariums
Wood Burning
Wooden Train Kit
Wreath Making
Yarn Picture

Self-esteem building

Bargello
Birdhouse Kit
Cinnamon Cut Outs
Collage
Counted Cross-Stitch Towel
Decoupage/Sponge Paint Flower Pot
Dough Art
Fly Tying
Jewelry
Latch Hook
Leather Moccasins Kit
Nail Art
Original Copper Tooling
Paper Twist Basket
Papier-Mâché
Pressed Flower Cards
Quilling
Rubbings
Snail Cribbage Board
Sponge-Stamped T-shirt
String Art
Terrariums
Wood Burning
Wooden Train Kit
Wreath Making
Yarn Picture

Release of negative feelings

Birdhouse Kit
Cinnamon Cut Outs
Dough Art
Nail Art
Needlepunch
Paper Making

Appendix E

Social Components

Responsibility

Needlepunch
Paper Making
String Art
Terrariums

Comfort level in group settings

Bargello
Birdhouse Kit
Cinnamon Cut Outs
Decoupage/Sponge Paint Flower Pot
Dough Art
Paper Making
Paper Twist Basket
Papier-Mâché
String Art
Wreath Making
Yarn Picture

Sociability with new situations

Bargello
Birdhouse Kit
Cinnamon Cut Outs
Dough Art
Paper Making
Paper Twist Basket
Papier-Mâché

Pressed Flower Cards
Wooden Train Kit
Yarn Picture

Ability to work alone

Bargello
Birdhouse Kit
Collage
Counted Cross-Stitch Towel
Decoupage/Sponge Paint Flower Pot
Dough Art
Fly Tying
Jewelry
Latch Hook
Leather Moccasins Kit
Nail Art
Needlepunch
Original Copper Tooling
Paper Making
Paper Twist Basket
Papier-Mâché
Pressed Flower Cards
Quilling
Rubbings
Snail Cribbage Board
Sponge-Stamped T-shirt
Terrariums
Wood Burning
Wooden Train Kit
Wreath Making
Yarn Picture

Appendix F

Adaptations

Position—sitting upright

Bargello
Birdhouse Kit
Cinnamon Cut Outs
Collage
Counted Cross-Stitch Towel
Decoupage/Sponge Paint Flower Pot
Dough Art
Fly Tying
Jewelry
Latch Hook
Leather Moccasins Kit
Nail Art
Needlepunch
Original Copper Tooling
Paper Making
Paper Twist Basket
Papier-Mâché
Pressed Flower Cards
Quilling
Rubbings
Snail Cribbage Board
Sponge-Stamped T-shirt
String Art
Terrariums
Wood Burning
Wooden Train Kit
Wreath Making
Yarn Picture

Position—reclined

Bargello
Collage
Counted Cross-Stitch Towel
Jewelry
Latch Hook
Leather Moccasins Kit
Needlepunch
Pressed Flower Cards
Quilling
String Art
Wooden Train Kit
Yarn Picture

Position—standing

Birdhouse Kit
Cinnamon Cut Outs
Collage
Decoupage/Sponge Paint Flower Pot
Dough Art
Nail Art
Paper Making
Papier-Mâché
Rubbings
Snail Cribbage Board
Sponge-Stamped T-shirt
Terrariums
Wreath Making

Allows for repetition of hand and finger motions

Bargello
Birdhouse Kit
Cinnamon Cut Outs
Counted Cross-Stitch Towel
Decoupage/Sponge Paint Flower Pot
Dough Art
Fly Tying

Jewelry
Latch Hook
Leather Moccasins Kit
Nail Art
Needlepunch
Original Copper Tooling
Paper Making
Paper Twist Basket
Papier-Mâché
Pressed Flower Cards
Quilling
Rubbings
String Art
Terrariums
Wood Burning
Wooden Train Kit
Wreath Making
Yarn Picture

For one-handed training with use of adaptive equipment

Bargello
Birdhouse Kit
Cinnamon Cut Outs
Collage
Counted Cross-Stitch Towel
Decoupage/Sponge Paint Flower Pot
Dough Art
Nail Art
Needlepunch
Original Copper Tooling
Paper Making
Papier-Mâché
Rubbings
Sponge-Stamped T-shirt
Wood Burning
Wreath Making
Yarn Picture

High success rate

Bargello
Birdhouse Kit
Cinnamon Cut Outs
Collage
Counted Cross-Stitch Towel
Decoupage/Sponge Paint Flower Pot
Dough Art
Jewelry
Latch Hook
Leather Moccasins Kit
Nail Art
Needlepunch
Paper Making
Paper Twist Basket
Papier-Mâché
Quilling
Sponge-Stamped T-shirt
Wooden Train Kit
Wreath Making
Yarn Picture

Can vary from a structured to an unstructured activity

Birdhouse Kit
Collage
Decoupage/Sponge Paint Flower Pot
Dough Art
Jewelry
Papier-Mâché
Pressed Flower Cards
Quilling
Rubbings
Sponge-Stamped T-shirt
Wreath Making

Can be done individually

- Bargello
- Birdhouse Kit
- Cinnamon Cut Outs
- Collage
- Counted Cross-Stitch Towel
- Decoupage/Sponge Paint Flower Pot
- Dough Art
- Fly Tying
- Jewelry
- Latch Hook
- Leather Moccasins Kit
- Nail Art
- Needlepunch
- Original Copper Tooling
- Paper Making
- Paper Twist Basket
- Papier-Mâché
- Quilling
- Rubbings
- Sponge-Stamped T-shirt
- String Art
- Terrariums
- Wood Burning
- Wooden Train Kit
- Wreath Making
- Yarn Picture

Design can incorporate some individual cultural values

- Collage
- Counted Cross-Stitch Towel
- Decoupage/Sponge Paint Flower Pot
- Dough Art
- Latch Hook
- Leather Moccasins Kit
- Nail Art
- Needlepunch

Original Copper Tooling
Quilling
Rubbings
Sponge-Stamped T-shirt
String Art
Terrariums
Wood Burning
Wreath Making
Yarn Picture

Appendix G

Miscellaneous Information

Crafts that provide olfactory stimulation

Cinnamon Cut Outs
Wood Burning

Crafts that could be used as safety/judgment evaluations for clients who would be returned to work

Snail Cribbage Board
Wood Burning

Crafts that could be used as a topographical orientation evaluation

Rubbings

Crafts appropriate for clients who are visually impaired

Cinnamon Cut Outs
Decoupage/Sponge Paint Flower Pot
Dough Art
Jewelry
Paper Twist Basket
Papier-Mâché
Quilling
Rubbings